ST. MARY'S HOSPITAL

Pharmacology Updates

Editor

JENNIFER WILBECK

NURSING CLINICS
OF NORTH AMERICA

www.nursing.theclinics.com

Consulting Editor
STEPHEN D. KRAU

March 2016 • Volume 51 • Number 1

ELSEVIER

1600 John F. Kennedy Boulevard • Suite 1800 • Philadelphia, Pennsylvania, 19103-2899

http://www.theclinics.com

NURSING CLINICS OF NORTH AMERICA Volume 51, Number 1
March 2016 ISSN 0029-6465, ISBN-13: 978-0-323-41653-5

Editor: Kerry Holland
Developmental Editor: Casey Jackson

Nursing Clinics of North America (ISSN 0029-6465) is published quarterly by Elsevier Inc., 360 Park Avenue South, New York, NY 10010-1710. Months of issue are March, June, September, and December. Periodicals postage paid at New York, NY and additional mailing offices. Subscription price per year is, $155.00 (US individuals), $447.00 (US institutions), $275.00 (international individuals), $545.00 (international institutions), $220.00 (Canadian individuals), $545.00 (Canadian institutions), $100.00 (US students), and $135.00 (international students). To receive student/resident rate, orders must be accompanied by name of affiliated institution, date of term, and the signature of program/residency coordinator on institution letterhead. Orders will be billed at individual rate until proof of status is received. Foreign air speed delivery is included in all *Clinics* subscription prices. All prices are subject to change without notice. **POSTMASTER:** Send address changes to *Nursing Clinics*, Elsevier Health Sciences Division, Subscription Customer Service, 3251 Riverport Lane, Maryland Heights, MO 63043. **Customer Service: Telephone: 1-800-654-2452** (U.S. and Canada); **1-314-447-8871 (outside U.S. and Canada). Fax: 1-314-447-8029. E-mail: journalscustomerservice-usa@elsevier.com** (for print support) and **journalsonlinesupport-usa@elsevier.com** (for online support).

Nursing Clinics of North America is covered in *EMBASE/Excerpta Medica, MEDLINE/PubMed (Index Medicus), Social Sciences Citation Index, Current Contents, ASCA, Cumulative Index to Nursing, RNdex Top 100,* and Allied Health Literature and International Nursing Index (INI).

Printed in the United States of America.

Contributors

CONSULTING EDITOR

STEPHEN D. KRAU, PhD, RN, CNE
Associate Professor, Vanderbilt University School of Nursing, Nashville, Tennessee

EDITOR

JENNIFER WILBECK, DNP, RN, ACNP-BC, FNP-BC
Associate Professor and ENP Specialty Director, Vanderbilt University School of Nursing, Nashville, Tennessee

AUTHORS

TERRI L. ALLISON, DNP, ACNP-BC, FAANP
Associate Professor of Nursing; Director, Doctor of Nursing Practice Program, Vanderbilt University School of Nursing, Nashville, Tennessee

CRAIG J. BEAVERS, PharmD, FAHA, AACC, BCPS-AQ Cardiology
CACP Clinical Pharmacy Coordinator, Cardiology and Cardiovascular Clinical Pharmacist Adjunct Faculty, Department of Pharmacy Practice and Science, University of Kentucky UK Healthcare, Lexington, Kentucky

MICHAEL D. GOOCH, MSN, ACNP-BC, FNP-BC, ENP-BC
Instructor in Nursing, Vanderbilt University School of Nursing, Nashville, Tennessee; Faculty, Middle Tennessee School of Anesthesia, Madison, Tennessee; Flight Nurse, Vanderbilt University Medical Center - LifeFlight, Nashville, Tennessee; Emergency Nurse Practitioner, TeamHealth at Maury Regional Medical Center, Columbia, Tennessee

MICHAEL D. HOGUE, PharmD, FAPhA, FNAP
Professor and Chair, Department of Pharmacy Practice, McWhorter School of Pharmacy, Samford University, Birmingham, Alabama

CAROLINE McGRATH, DNP, CRNA
Colonel, United States Air Force; Adjunct Faculty, Vanderbilt University School of Nursing, Nashville, Tennessee

ANNA E. MEADOR, PharmD, BCACP
Assistant Professor of Pharmacy Practice, Pharmacy Director, Christ Health Center; McWhorter School of Pharmacy, Samford University, Birmingham, Alabama

SHEILA MELANDER, PhD, ACNP-BC, FCCM, FAANP
Assistant Dean of Graduate Faculty Affairs, Director of the DNP/MSN Program, Norton's Healthcare System, University of Kentucky, Owensboro, Kentucky

STEPHEN MILLER, ANP, MSN, ACNP-BC
Adjunct faculty, Vanderbilt School of Nursing; Tennova Turkey Creek Medical Center, Knoxville, Tennessee

KOMAL A. PANDYA, PharmD, BCPS
Cardiothoracic Surgery Clinical Pharmacy Specialist Adjunct Faculty, Department of Pharmacy Practice and Science, University of Kentucky UK Healthcare, Lexington, Kentucky

ERIC ROBERTS, DNP, FNP-BC, ENP-BC
Assistant Professor, Loyola University Chicago, Marcella Neihoff School of Nursing, Maywood, Illinois

MEGAN M. SHIFRIN, DNP, RN, ACNP-BC
Vanderbilt University School of Nursing, Nashville, Tennessee

JULIE STEPHENS, PharmD, BCPS
Assistant Professor of Pharmacy Practice, Lipscomb University College of Pharmacy, Nashville, Tennessee

S. BRIAN WIDMAR, PhD, RN, ACNP-BC, CCRN
Vanderbilt University School of Nursing, Nashville, Tennessee

CHRISTOPHER TY WILLIAMS, DNP, RN, ACNP-BC, FNP-BC
Instructor in Nursing, DNP Program, Vanderbilt University School of Nursing, Nashville, Tennessee

MICHAEL WRIGHT, PharmD, BCPS
Critical Care Clinical Specialist, Department of Pharmacy, Williamson Medical Center, Franklin, Tennessee

COURTNEY J. YOUNG, DNP, MPH, FNP-BC
Assistant Professor, Vanderbilt University School of Nursing, Nashville, Tennessee

Contents

> In this article, the processing of investigational and new drug applications is described and the standard and expedited review processes are examined. The efforts of the US Food and Drug Administration to ensure greater agency transparency and fiscal responsibility and intensify oversight during the drug development and approval process are reviewed. Often attributed to a decrease in the number of uninsured adults, both the increase in prescription drug sales and the high costs associated with bringing a new drug to market highlight the necessity for a streamlined and cost-effective process to deliver these drugs safely and effectively.

> Treatment options for patients with heart failure (HF) have improved in recent years. Medication combinations along with improved device management have improved survival rates and quality of life for patients with HF. Most patients with HF are older than 65 years. Because patients with HF with multiple comorbidities and any physical or cognitive impairments are often excluded from trials or studies, the evidence to guide therapy for most older patients with HF is not always representative and requires customization. Health care providers must remember that older patients with HF with multiple comorbidities and polypharmacy are at great risk for adverse effects and drug-to-drug interactions.

> Antithrombotic medications have become standard of care for management of acute coronary syndrome. Platelet adhesion, activation, and aggregation are essential components of platelet function; platelet-inhibiting medications interfere with these components and reduce incidence of thrombosis. Active bleeding is a contraindication for administration of platelet inhibitors. There is currently no reversal agent for platelet inhibitors, although platelet transfusion may be used to correct active bleeding after administration of platelet inhibitors.

Human immunodeficiency virus has been affecting the human population for more than 30 years. During this time period, more effective, safe, simple, and tolerable pharmacologic agents have been developed. To date, there are 26 antiretroviral agents available that are used either as a single agent or a coformulation in an antiretroviral regimen. The goal of these medications is to achieve viral suppression in individuals infected with human immunodeficiency virus. Evidence continues to support the most effective combinations. It is important that clinicians are knowledgeable of updates so as to provide the best possible medical regimen for this population.

Poisoning is the leading cause of injury-related mortality in the United States. Data suggest that nonmedical use of pharmaceuticals is increasing, along with a proportional increase in subsequent adverse events. The widespread use of illegal drugs contributes to the challenge, because these drugs may produce a wide array of clinical presentations that warrant time-critical recognition and treatment. Common legal and illegal poisonings highlighting clinical presentations in terms of toxidromes as a means of categorically recognizing these emergencies is the focus of this article. To optimize outcomes for situations such as these, pharmacologic considerations are discussed and explored.

Health care providers should be aware of the pharmacotherapy considerations in the American Heart Association's guidelines for advanced cardiac life support (ACLS). Current evidence does not suggest a reduction in mortality with ACLS medications; however, these medications can improve return of spontaneous circulation. Proper agent selection and dosing are imperative to maximize benefit and minimize harm. The latest guideline update included major changes to the ventricular fibrillation/pulseless ventricular tachycardia and pulseless electrical activity/asystole algorithms, which providers should adopt. It is critical that providers be prepared for post-code management. Health care professionals should remain abreast of changing evidence and guidelines.

Massive transfusion practices were transformed during the 1970s without solid evidence supporting the use of component therapy. A manual literature search was performed for all references to the lethal triad, acute or early coagulopathy of trauma, fresh whole blood, and component transfusion therapy in massive trauma, and damage control resuscitation. Data from recent wars suggest traditional component therapy causes a nonhemostatic resuscitation worsening the propagation of the lethal triad hastening death. These same studies also indicate the advantage of fresh whole blood over component therapy even when administered in a 1:1:1 replacement ratio.

Pain and agitation may be difficult to assess in a critically ill patient. Pain is best assessed by self-reporting pain scales; but in patients who are unable to communicate, behavioral pain scales seem to have benefit. Patients' sedation level should be assessed each shift and preferably by a validated ICU tool, such as the RASS or SAS scale. Pain is most appropriately treated with the use of opiates, and careful consideration should be given to the pharmacokinetic and pharmacodynamic properties of various analgesics to determine the optimal agent for each individual patient. Sedation levels should preferably remain light or with the use of a daily awakening trial. Preferred treatment of agitation is analgosedation with the addition of nonbenzodiazepine sedatives if necessary. There are risks associated with each agent used in the treatment of pain and agitation, and it is important to monitor patients for effectiveness, signs of toxicity, and adverse drug reactions.

This article discusses immunosuppressive medications used in organ and hematopoietic stem cell transplantation. Induction, maintenance, and rescue therapy are administered throughout different periods during and after transplantation to modulate the immune system response in the recipient to prevent or treat rejection or graft-versus-host disease. Indications, dosing strategies, required monitoring, complications, adverse events, and concomitant drug interactions associated with immunosuppressive medications are presented. Classes of medications discussed include polyclonal and monoclonal antibodies, calcineurin inhibitors, antiproliferative agents, mammalian target of rapamycin inhibitors, and corticosteroids. Medications having significant interactions with immunosuppression are also examined.

Vaccines are among most cost-effective public health strategies. Despite effective vaccines for many bacterial and viral illnesses, tens of thousands of adults and hundreds of children die each year in the United States from vaccine-preventable diseases. Underutilization of vaccines requires rethinking the approach to incorporating vaccines into practice. Arguably, immunizations could be a part all health care encounters. Shared responsibility is paramount if deaths are to be reduced. This article reviews the available vaccines in the US market, as well as practice recommendations of the Centers for Disease Control and Prevention's Advisory Committee on Immunization Practices.

NURSING CLINICS OF NORTH AMERICA

Foreword

The Role of Pharmacogenomics: The Same Medications Do Not Work the Same on Everyone

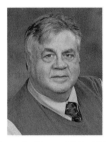

Stephen D. Krau, PhD, RN, CNE
Consulting Editor

The scope of pharmacology and all dimensions of pharmacology are rapidly expanding. This focuses the nurse's attention to not only the new medications and their effects on patients, but also how to better predict and monitor outcomes. Currently much prescribing involves primary care provider decision-making coupled with the traditional "trial and error."[1] In this decision process, prescribers consider such factors as FDA approvals and warnings, patient's previous treatments, the patient's presenting symptoms, practice guidelines, and patient preferences.

Over time, the prescriber becomes comfortable with the use of certain medications in his or her practice and has gained personal knowledge about certain medications through experience. There follows a tendency to prescribe similar medications without true consideration for individual variations and phenotyping among patients.[2] This results in an "experiment" each time a new medication is prescribed for a patient. The nurse administering the medication becomes the judge for the "trial" as well as the judge for the potential "error." Although the medication is FDA approved, it is well-known that due to variant phenotypes, including gender, the same medications do not work the same on everyone. For example, it is known that the incidence of myocardial infarction among women is less than that for men; however, the mortality for women who experience myocardial infarctions is disproportionately higher. One need only look at the evidence as to the variations among symptoms between men and women, and the population (or in this case gender) that provides the basis for diagnosis. One need only look at the populations that were involved in drug testing to know that an adverse effect is more likely in populations not considered in the clinical drug trials of the medications. Although we administer medications to many of the same patients, one phenotype does not "fit" all patients. This can result in overmedicating, undermedicating, or even medicating the patient with the wrong medication. It is the

http://dx.doi.org/10.1016/j.cnur.2015.12.002
0029-6465/16/$ – see front matter © 2016 Published by Elsevier Inc.
nursing.theclinics.com

responsibility of the nurse to monitor for, and report any adverse effects the patient experiences due to the effect of medications.

Given the high risk associated with medication administration and prescribing, the nurse becomes the pivotal constant in treatments involving medications. As such, safe practice can only occur when the nurse has the skill set and knowledge to evaluate different medications and understand what influences different outcomes. It has taken decades for the science related to cytochrome p450 to reach clinical practice. Nurse understanding of the metabolic activities of this classification of enzymes on drug metabolism is an essential part of the nurse's role as "judge" during the trial and potential for error when drugs new to the patient are administered. Understanding the metabolic effects of these enzymes that breaks down more than 30 classes of drugs and 60% to 80% of the most commonly prescribed drugs is essential.[3]

Each time a nurse tells a patient to avoid taking grapefruit juice with a certain medication, cytochrome p450 provides the basis. Grapefruit juice is metabolized by the same cytochrome p450 as many medications. As such, grapefruit juice inhibits the metabolization of many medications, which can lead to toxic effects. Even without knowing the rationale for cautioning a patient about grapefruit juice, the nurse is using evidence that has been discovered related to cytochrome p450. So, the incremental advances of knowledge in this area have been considered in clinical practice, but without a solid knowledge base for the nurse that explains certain recommendations.[3]

Amounts of different cytochrome p450 enzymes vary from person to person based on his or her phenotype. This makes drug metabolism and effect somewhat unpredictable when the medication is new for the patient.

The nurse, in collaboration with the patient, provides the data for determining the effective and safe use of medications that are new for the patient. The more the nurse knows, or more information that is provided the patient, the safer the situation. It is imperative that nurses engage in "lifelong" learning about medications and also the many new medications that are approved annually. For this learning to be effective and integrate to clinical practice, the nurse should become familiar with terms and concepts used in genetics and pharmacogenetics. This understanding will improve patient safety as the nurse evaluates, "judges," and reports the impact of genetics on patient outcomes related to drug therapy.

Stephen D. Krau, PhD, RN, CNE
Vanderbilt University School of Nursing
461 21st Avenue South
Nashville, TN, 37202, USA

E-mail address:
steve.krau@vanderbilt.edu

REFERENCES

1. Turner RM. From the lab to prescription pad: genetics, CYP450 analysis, and medication response. J Child Adolesc Psychiatr Nurs 2013;26:119–23.
2. Hall-Flavin DK, SchneeKloth TD, Allen JD. Translational psychiatry: bringing pharmacogenomics testing into clinical practice. Prim Psychiatry 2010;17(5):39–44.
3. Krau SD. Cytochrome p450 part 3: drug interactions: essential concepts and considerations. Nurs Clin North Am 2013;48(4):697–706.

Preface

Pharmacologic Therapies: An Enduring Nursing Intervention

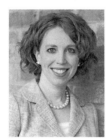

Jennifer Wilbeck, DNP, RN, ACNP-BC, FNP-BC
Editor

From the earliest days of nursing as a profession, administration of medications has been recognized as an integral part of the professional role. In less than ideal circumstances, and with little (if any) scientific understanding of cellular physiology, Florence Nightingale provided medicines to soldiers in attempts to ward off diseases, promote healing, and provide comfort. More than 150 years later, in light of scientific advances and evolution of the professional role, nurses today continue providing medications to promote healing and comfort as Nightingale did during the Crimean War.

In fact, much of recent medical discovery is rooted in research utilizing data obtained in a theater of war. In her article exploring the use of blood and blood products, McGrath details how data collected from casualties of modern wars provide the evidence to support updated practice recommendations regarding component blood therapy. Translation of new evidence, be it garnered from a war zone or clinical lab, is ultimately converted into new pharmacologic therapies following a prescribed process outlined in Williams' article on the FDA process of pharmaceutical regulation.

Much like the growth of scientific discoveries and medication production, the opportunities and settings for nursing practice have exponentially expanded in past years. While at first glance the topics contained within this issue may appear exceptionally broad, they in fact represent issues congruent with the diversity of our nursing practice. Increasingly complex care is now routinely delivered in outpatient arenas. Diagnoses once considered to be life-threatening (such as HIV infection) may now represent a chronic medical condition. Furthermore, issues that were once isolated to specialty areas of nursing, such as pediatrics or transplant, now represent routine encounters for nurses across all specialty areas.

Accordingly, this issue was designed in the hopes of offering something for all nurses regardless of practice setting. It is my hope that as you read this issue, there will be some information that you can apply to your practice today. I hope that you will uncover something in the following pages that strengthens you as a patient advocate,

Nurs Clin N Am 51 (2016) xi–xii
http://dx.doi.org/10.1016/j.cnur.2015.12.001
0029-6465/16/$ – see front matter **nursing.theclinics.com**

that prepares you to anticipate a complication, or that allows you to provide better treatment or comfort. After all, it's what we do!

Jennifer Wilbeck, DNP, RN, ACNP-BC, FNP-BC
Vanderbilt University School of Nursing
461 21st Avenue South, 336 Frist Hall
Nashville, TN 37240, USA

E-mail address:
jennifer.wilbeck@vanderbilt.edu

Food and Drug Administration Drug Approval Process
A History and Overview

Christopher Ty Williams, DNP, RN, ACNP-BC, FNP-BC

KEYWORDS

- Food and Drug Administration • Drug review • Drug approval • Expedited reviews

KEY POINTS

- The US Food and Drug Administration (FDA) is a science-based regulatory agency with a public health mission, including the review and surveillance of human and veterinary drugs.
- Before filing a new drug application, 3 phases of investigational clinical trials must be completed. Typically, at least 2 phase 3 clinical trials are required.
- The length of time required to complete preclinical and clinical testing can be 10 to 15 years.
- Decreasing numbers of uninsured Americans and escalating development costs highlight the need to bring drugs to market in a safe, expeditious manner.

INTRODUCTION

From 2010 to mid-2014, the number of uninsured working-aged adults decreased by 16%, or 8 million people.[1] This reduction was associated with the increased availability of subsidized insurance options. Furthermore, working-aged adults have reported increased access to care and decreased stress linked to insurance-related financial burdens.[1] Representing an increase of 12.2% from the previous period, US prescription sales for the period October, 2013 to September, 2014 totaled $360.7 billion dollars.[2] This increase was attributed to the improving US economy and the increased number of individuals who gained insurance through the provisions of the Patient Protection and Affordable Care Act (PPACA) of 2010. In 2015, overall health care spending is estimated to increase 17.6%.[2]

As of 2014, the cost of bringing a new drug to market in the United States can exceed $2.5 billion.[3,4] In an effort to meet consumer and industry demands, the US

Disclosure: The author declares that there are no conflicts of interest.
DNP Program, Vanderbilt University School of Nursing, 461 21st Avenue South, Nashville, TN 37240, USA
E-mail address: christopher.t.williams@vanderbilt.edu

Food and Drug Administration (FDA) has taken efforts to streamline the new drug testing and approval process, including shortening the median approval time for new drugs from 19 to 10 months.[3] In 2011, the FDA approved 30 new therapeutics (molecular entities and biologics), the most since 2004. Approved drugs consisted of 11 first-in-class agents, including drugs developed to treat unaddressed diseases and to reach new populations.[5] The purpose of this article is to review the FDA's history and milestone legislation and to provide an overview of the FDA's drug development and approval processes.

BACKGROUND

The FDA operates within the US Department of Health and Human Services as a "science-based regulatory agency with a public health mission."[3,6] The FDA has multiple missions, including ensuring public health through monitoring the safety and efficacy of human and veterinary drugs and devices (brand name and generic), as well as developing strategies to increase both safety and efficacy.[6,7] The FDA is also responsible for monitoring and ensuring the safety of foods and cosmetics, including production in sanitary conditions and the use of safe ingredients.[3,6] In addition, tobacco products fall under the jurisdiction of the FDA, which also advocates for smoking cessation and reducing the number of minors who consume tobacco products. The FDA is charged with ensuring the safety of vaccines, biopharmaceuticals, blood products, medical devices, and electromagnetic radiation-emitting devices. Current strategic priorities for the organization, as directed by Congress, include safety and quality, regulatory science, smart regulation, globalization, and stewardship.[6]

Concepts

Safety, efficacy, and effectiveness are key concepts involved in understanding the FDA drug development and approval process. Safety can be measured by evaluating adverse reactions related to drug exposure or by toxicity testing, when the highest tolerable or optimal dose is determined.[8] Efficacy refers to the performance of the drug compared with placebo in a near-ideal environment, such as a clinical trial, in which investigators can control conditions. Similarly, effectiveness provides a real-life description of the action of the drug, which can be affected by comorbidities, medication interactions, and other wide-ranging factors and variables.[8]

Prescription drug labeling information is also commonly known as prescribing information or package inserts. Drug labels are required to provide a summary of safe and effective drug use. They are required to be accurate, with no false or misleading statements or implied claims.[9,10] Although patients may benefit from drug labeling, its primary purpose is to give health care providers the essential information needed to appropriately prescribe the drug.[10]

Importantly, drug labeling does not substitute for FDA-approved patient education materials. In 2006, the FDA reformatted drug-labeling requirements, with input from focus groups, surveys, and public meetings with prescribers.[9] The revision added specific sections (eg, highlights of prescribing information) and reordered and reorganized other sections for clarity and completeness. The adverse reactions section consolidated all risk information and, in efforts to encourage adverse event reporting, includes the telephone number and Web address for the manufacturer and MedWatch, the FDA's adverse reporting system. Furthermore, the adverse reactions from clinical trials are reported separately from postmarket surveillance. Since 2006, all new drug applications (NDAs) must conform to FDA labeling requirements at the time of submission.[9,10]

Center for Drug Evaluation and Research

The Center for Drug Evaluation and Research (CDER) is the largest of the FDA's 6 centers. Considered to be a watchdog for consumers, the CDER's main purpose is to evaluate the safety, efficacy, and risks of all new brand name and generic drugs.[3,11,12] Since the FDA's 2002 *Pharmaceutical Current Good Manufacturing Practices for the 21st Century* initiative, the CDER has actively promoted quality measures to modernize human and veterinary drug regulation policies and procedures.[12] Strategies include encouraging early adoption of technology and enhancing the FDA's business processes and regulatory policies. However, increasing drug shortages (including sterile injectable drugs, orphan drugs, and oncology drugs) led to an executive order in October, 2011 that expanded the CDER's authority in containing drug shortages.

Within the CDER, the Office of New Drugs has regulatory oversight for investigational studies and makes marketing decisions for new and existing drugs. In January, 2015, the FDA restructured CDER to include the new Office of Pharmaceutical Quality (OPQ). The OPQ is intended to improve oversight of the quality of a drug throughout the life cycle of the product. Furthermore, the office realigns agency resources to create 1 consistent program for new, brand name, generic, over-the-counter (OTC), and prescription drugs.[13]

Code of Federal Regulations

The Code of Federal Regulations (CFR) Title 21 established an efficient and thorough drug review process, facilitating approval of drugs with proven safety and efficacy.[14] The CFR described the submission requirements and outlined the procedures by which the FDA evaluates, approves, and monitors new drugs, including amendments, supplements, and postmarket reporting.[14] Furthermore, the CFR blocks the FDA from rejecting an NDA based on efficacy of questionable clinical significance, provided the new drug showed a statistically significant result compared with placebo.[15]

HISTORY

From its origins in 1848, the FDA became a federal consumer protection agency after the US Congress's passage of the Pure Food and Drugs Act of 1906. The focus of the Act was labeling, rather than evaluating, the safety of a drug.[16,17] The public's concern about the safety of OTC and prescription drugs intensified during the New Deal period, particularly after the deaths of 100 adults and children who used Massengill's elixir sulfanilamide in 1937.[17,18] Subsequently, the regulatory authority of the FDA was expanded with Congress's passage of the Federal Food, Drug, and Cosmetic Act (FFDCA) of 1938.

The FFDCA empowered the FDA to review the manufacturer's evidence that the drug was safe. The FFDCA banned false claims by drug manufacturers and, for the first time, required that manufacturers file an NDA. However, an NDA was automatically approved if the FDA did not meet the burden of proving that the drug was unsafe. Furthermore, the FFDCA expanded educational efforts, focusing on elimination of misbranding, safe medication use, and providing consumers with scientifically sound information.[3,19] Unexpectedly, the FFDCA also resulted in unclear legal distinctions between OTC and prescription drugs.[18]

The Durham-Humphrey Amendment of 1951 clarified the legal distinction among OTC and prescription drugs and created a process for the FDA to categorize drugs.[16] In 1961, thalidomide, a non–FDA-approved sedative used to treat morning sickness in pregnant women, was pulled from the market after being linked to birth defects, spurring public attention worldwide. Subsequently, passage of the Kefauver-Harris Amendment, also known as the Drug Efficacy Amendment, expanded the FDA's role in 1962, mandating that new drugs be tested for safety and requiring applicants to prove efficacy and disclose adverse effects before marketing.[11,17] Pursuant to this amendment, all drugs that were on the market were evaluated and classified by the Drug Efficacy Study Implementation program as effective, ineffective, or needing further study.

Amendments to the FFDCA continued over the next 30 years. For instance, the 1983 Orphan Drug Act and the 1984 Hatch-Waxman Act incentivized pharmaceutical manufacturers to develop drugs for rare diseases and increased access to lower-cost generic drugs, respectively.[20] As a result of intense regulation, lack of FDA resources, increased consumer demand, and rapid pharmaceutical drug development, applicants faced significant delays in drug approval, which frustrated consumers, pharmaceutical manufacturers, and the FDA.[11,20]

In 1992, Congress passed the Prescription Drug User Fee Act (PDUFA), modifying the FFDCA and allowing drug manufacturers themselves to fund the FDA drug approval process by contributing to the FDA's resources.[20] The PDUFA also instituted goals for timelier drug approvals and established standards and timelines for completion of NDA reviews. In addition, the PDUFA paved the way for the FDA to allow drug manufacturers to market drugs before approval, if testing was completed while the drug was on the market. Since 1992, more than 1000 drugs and biologics have received FDA approval.[11,20]

The 1997 FDA Modernization Act also amended the FFDCA and re-extended the PDUFA. Clinical testing requirements were modified, access to experimental therapies was increased, and advertising off-label drug use was no longer prohibited.[20,21] Pediatric testing was finally regulated via the 2002 Best Pharmaceuticals for Children Act (BPCA) and the 2003 Pediatric Research Equity Act (PREA), which required pediatric drug assessments to be included in NDAs.[11,20] Congress has further amended the FFDCA in recent years through passage of the Family Smoking Prevention and Tobacco Control Act of 2009, the PPACA of 2010, and the Drug Quality and Security Act of 2013.[6,19,20,22]

The FDA Safety and Innovation Act of 2013 (FDASIA), also known as the User Fee Reauthorization Act, continued and expanded the FDA's practice of collecting fees from applicants to fund testing of generic drugs, innovator or specialty drugs for new diseases, medical devices, and biosimilar biological products.[23] Specialty drugs, those targeted at specific diseases or populations, including orphan (underdeveloped), oncology and obesity drugs, have been identified as driving the increase in prescription drug expenditures in 2014, with a further expected increase in 2015.[2,5,23] The FDASIA also expanded the role of clinicians and patients throughout the development process and empowered the FDA to designate drugs as breakthrough therapy, qualifying them for expedited development and review. The FDASIA intensified the focus on pediatric drug development by making permanent the PREA, BPCA, and the Pediatric Medical Device Quality Act.[3,19,23]

DRUG DEVELOPMENT AND APPROVAL PROCESS

The development process for new drugs is divided into 2 sections (preclinical and clinical) and typically spans 12 to 15 years, excluding postmarket surveillance throughout the lifetime of the drug (**Fig. 1**).[3,20] Rigorous preclinical laboratory testing (including animal studies) assesses the biological activity and safety of a new drug and, on average, takes 5.5 years to complete. Approximately 5 of 5000 new drugs complete the preclinical phase and advance to clinical trials in humans. Of those 5, 1 drug is typically approved by the FDA and reaches the marketplace.[24] Before marketing a new drug, pharmaceutical

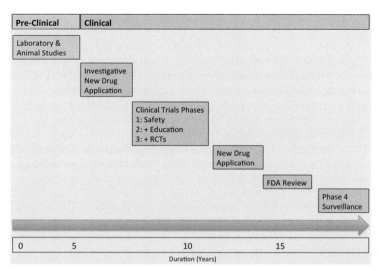

Fig. 1. Standard drug development and approval process. RCT, randomized controlled trial.

sponsors must complete the 4 steps outlined by the FDA: investigational new drug (IND) application, clinical trials, NDA, and FDA review (standard or expedited).[3,20]

Investigational New Drug Application

The drug sponsor, based on promising evidence from preclinical laboratory studies, submits an IND application describing the prospective study to the CDER.[3,12,24] The IND application presents information on animal pharmacology and toxicology, chemistry, manufacturing, and clinical protocols. Institutional Review Board (IRB) approval is included, which details the proposed plan for protection of human participants, including informed consent language and a statement of risks.[3,14] The applicants must specify the indication for use, noting the mechanism of action, clinical condition, and intended population of the drug. An FDA review board examines the IND for scientific validity and ethical implications within 30 days of submission. Barring any objections, the applicant may begin clinical trials immediately after FDA approval of the IND application.[3,14,24]

Clinical Trials

Building on the safety shown in animal trials and laboratory studies, clinical trials test safety and efficacy of drugs in volunteer human participants and investigate any previously undocumented adverse reactions.[20,24] Clinical trials help determine whether new drugs should be approved for use in the general population. The FDA's Office of Good Clinical Practice and Human Subject Protection coordinates the FDA's Bioresearch Monitoring program that oversees, advises on, and assists with issues arising from clinical trials, particularly those involving human participants. The FDA retains the right to issue a clinical hold or interrupt a clinical trial at any time.[20,24]

Clinical trials of new drugs are designated sequentially. Phases 1, 2, and 3 are conducted before submitting an NDA, whereas phase 4 studies are conducted after market, after the approval and release of the drug.[3,20] Phase 1 studies focus on safety, frequently using a single-blind study design. They are designed to determine drug dosing, identify the most frequent side effects of a drug, measure the kinetic activity (metabolism and excretion) of a drug, and, most importantly, minimize risk to human participants. Infrequently, these studies may yield evidence of drug efficacy. The sample for a phase 1 clinical trial typically consists of 20 to 80 healthy volunteers and the phase lasts 2 years on average.[3,20,24]

Phase 2 studies emphasize efficacy, continue to monitor safety, and seek preliminary data (eg, effective doses) based on a specific disease within an identified population. These studies identify short-term, common side effects. Phase 2 studies use a control group and the number of participants typically ranges from 100 to 300 patients. The average study duration is 2 years. After phase 2, the FDA and drug sponsors collaborate on phase 3 study designs.[3,20,24]

Phase 3 studies are used to confirm the efficacy and validate the safety findings of previous studies in a larger population, using randomized clinical trials. Phase 3 studies evaluate diverse populations, drug dosages, and the use of the drug in combination with other pharmaceuticals. These studies also monitor for adverse events related to long-term use. The number of participants ranges from several hundred to 3000 patient volunteers. The average phase 3 duration is 2 to 4 years.[3,20,24]

New Drug Application

After the successful completion of clinical trials, a drug manufacturer or sponsor may submit an NDA to the CDER. The NDA is a formal request for the FDA to evaluate the safety of a drug and approve it for sale in the United States. The NDA presents complete information on the chemical formula, specifications, pharmacodynamics, and pharmacokinetics of a drug.[20,24] In addition, pharmacometric analysis has come to play an important role in the NDA review process, affecting decisions related to trial design, labeling, and drug approval.[25] The NDA also includes indications for use (including disease and population), labeling information, preclinical and animal testing results, clinical trial results, and manufacturing data, including quality control and assurance procedures.[3,20] Once accepted, an NDA undergoes an extensive review process by the CDER to validate the sponsors' assertions and findings.

Standard Reviews

After submission of an NDA, the CDER has 60 days to file the application for review. A trained review team of physicians, chemists, microbiologists, pharmacologists, statisticians, and other experts convene to evaluate the safety of the new drug and to validate previous findings. Before 1992, there were reports of NDA reviews lasting 2 to 3 years. Per the PDUFA, the CDER is now expected to review and act on at least 90% of NDAs within 10 months for standard drugs, and priority drugs should be reviewed within 6 months. These goals serve as justification for allowing drug sponsors to pay for fees associated with FDA review processes.[3,20,24,26]

The FDA review team considers 3 issues when reviewing an NDA:

- "Whether the drug is safe and effective in its proposed use, and whether the benefits of the drug outweigh its risks
- Whether the drug's proposed labeling (package insert) is appropriate, and what it should contain
- Whether the methods used to manufacture the drug and the controls used to maintain the drug's quality are adequate to preserve the drug's identity, strength, quality and purity"[20]

FDA scientific and regulatory personnel evaluate the following categories: medical, pharmacology, chemistry, biopharmaceutical, clinical, statistical, risk assessment and mitigation, proprietary name, and label and labeling. The FFDCA requires "substantial evidence" of drug safety and effectiveness, which is interpreted to require that the drug manufacturer or sponsor provides evidence from at least 2 phase 3 studies demonstrating effectiveness.[3,20] If needed, the CDER may assemble an advisory panel of subject-matter experts, patient group leaders, and industry representatives to make recommendations on the approvability of the application. Most often, these panels are assembled to address drugs with new pharmacologic actions or significant safety risks.[3,20,24]

Based on the review of evidence, the FDA can approve an NDA with or without specific conditions or restrictions. After approval, the FDA sends the applicant a complete response letter. Previously, approvable and not approvable letters were sent.[20] Commonly, an NDA approval includes clinical and nonclinical postmarket commitments to ensure ongoing safety and effectiveness within special populations and to develop strategies to minimize inappropriate use of the drug.[3]

The response letter for rejected applications identifies deficiencies and includes specific recommendations for improvement. Common reasons for rejection of an NDA include issues with the clinical evidence of safety and effectiveness of a drug, as well as problems with manufacturing controls, labeling, human participant protection, and patent information.[9] If rejected, an applicant's recourse includes withdrawing the NDA, resubmitting additional data addressing identified deficiencies, and requesting a hearing with the CDER.[3,20]

The FDA's Division of Scientific Investigations (DSI) is charged with maintaining the quality of clinical data and protecting the rights of participants in clinical trials. The DSI inspects clinical study sites and reviews IRB records to ensure patient protection. Furthermore, it evaluates use of the proper inclusion and exclusion criteria for the sample, whether studies were conducted per the established investigational plan, and whether all adverse events were reported (FDA's drug review process). The CDER conducts close to 400 clinical investigator inspections annually, of which 3% are classified "official action indicated."[20,24]

Expedited Review

The FDA has established 4 mechanisms to facilitate drug development and review: fast-track, breakthrough therapy, accelerated approval, and priority review.[26] The fast-track process was designed to facilitate and expedite the development and review of drugs that were developed to treat serious medical conditions and fill an unmet medical need. Severity is determined based on the impact of the drug on activities of daily living and its ability to prevent disease progression. Unmet medical needs are defined as diseases or conditions with no current therapy; if available therapies exist, a fast-track drug must show a relative advantage, such as superior effectiveness, decreased toxicity, improved diagnosis and outcomes, or the ability to address an anticipated or emerging public health need. Requests for fast-track designation can be filed at any time during drug development, and the FDA response time is 60 days.[26]

The designation of breakthrough therapy is intended to expedite development and review (in the same manner as fast-track) of a new drug targeting a serious condition in which preliminary clinical evidence about the new drug indicates a potential improvement over the available therapy.[26] The drug sponsor or manufacturer may request breakthrough therapy status, typically no later than the end of phase 2, and before submission of an NDA. As with the fast-track application, the FDA processes breakthrough therapy requests within 60 days of receipt.

The accelerated approval regulations were developed based on the awareness that measuring the positive therapeutic effect, or clinical benefit, of a new drug can take an extended period. These regulations established that drugs fulfilling an unmet medical need can be approved based on the use of a surrogate end point, expediting FDA approval. Many anti–human immunodeficiency virus drugs, for example, have been approved via the accelerated approval route in which a surrogate end point acts as a predictor, rather than a measure, of clinical benefit. Examples of surrogate end points include data based on laboratory values, radiographic images, and physical signs. Studies using surrogate end points must be "adequate and well controlled" per the FFDCA.[20,26] Once a drug is approved, drug manufacturers must confirm the initial results or risk losing FDA approval.

Unlike other forms of expedited review, the priority review process, as established under the PDUFA, does not begin until after an NDA has been submitted. The goal of a priority review designation is for the FDA to take action on an application within 6 months, compared with 10 months for a standard NDA. Furthermore, a priority review directs attention to drugs that could represent significant improvements in the safety or effectiveness of the treatment, diagnosis, or prevention of serious conditions when compared with standard applications.[26] Although not explicitly required by law, the FDA's current practice is to assign priority review status to any drug that addresses an unmet need. The designation of priority status has no effect on the duration of clinical trial phases, nor does it affect the scientific and medical standard to which studies are held.

Phase 4 Surveillance

Once a drug is approved, the postmarketing monitoring stage begins. Phase 4 surveillance studies monitor the safety and real-world effectiveness of a drug to ensure optimal use after release into the marketplace. Phase 4 surveillance can include non-interventional studies, large simple trials, postmarketing surveillance studies, adverse event monitoring, case-control studies, drug utilization studies, and prospective observational studies, such as registries.[20,27] Because the drug approval process is based primarily on results of clinical trials, in which small samples are selected with strict inclusion and exclusion criteria, increased vigilance during this phase is necessary to ensure that the long-term benefits of a drug outweigh identified risks.

Although phase 1 to 3 clinical trials are unlikely to detect adverse reactions that occur in fewer than 3000 to 5000 patients, phase 4 studies are more likely to detect adverse reactions because of the larger population and presence of comorbidities.[20,27] Phase 4 surveillance continues as long as the drug is on the market. When the FDA is notified of a change in the safety profile of an approved drug, risk is assessed and managed. This assessment may be accomplished by changes to drug labeling, implementation of a risk management program, black box warnings, or withdrawing the drug from the market.[11]

Calls from the Institute of Medicine (IOM) to improve the drug regulation system in the United States have heightened postmarket surveillance efforts. The FDA implemented Risk Evaluation and Mitigation Strategies (REMS), previously known as Risk Minimization Action Plans (RiskMAPS), to show its commitment to enhancing patient safety.[28,29] REMS consist of at least 1 of 3 components: an FDA-approved Medication Guide, a Communication Plan, and Elements to Assure Safe Use. However, few data describing existing REMS are available to support their continued use.[28] More recently, the IOM has called for the FDA to restructure postmarket surveillance efforts to require real-time data reporting of early signs of drug toxicity.[3]

CRITICISM AND CONTROVERSY

Although the FDA has addressed concerns related to the lengthy development and review process and the lack of research into the safety and efficacy of pediatric medications, criticisms and controversy remain related to the drug approval process. The FDA has been accused of being overly hasty in the review and approval process. Other critics have called the FDA risk averse, slow, and inefficient, especially compared with the European Union (EU).[30] However, few data exist to confirm either of these criticisms. A review of new oncology drugs during the period 2003 to 2010 showed a median approval time of 6 months, consistent with expedited review goals. Furthermore, the new oncology drugs became available to patients in the United States sooner than they were available to patients in the EU.[3,30]

Claims of FDA bias toward drug manufacturers have frequently been related to the continued practice of collecting user fees, paid by drug manufacturers or sponsors to support the drug approval process. Some argue that this requirement biases the FDA review in favor of the drug sponsor. Over the past decade, after market withdrawals related to concerns about pharmaceutical safety and effectiveness, specifically of drugs used primarily for gastroenterology, diabetes, and musculoskeletal pain, significant controversy was generated calling into question the rigor of the drug review process.[3] To address concerns, the FDA OPQ has developed policies and procedures designed to safeguard clinical performance; enhance science-based and risk-based regulatory approaches; transform product oversight into a quantitative and expertise-based assessment; seamlessly integrate review, inspection, surveillance, and policy across the market life span of a drug; and encourage the exploration and integration of emerging pharmaceutical technology.[13]

In 2008, York University[31] estimated that US pharmaceutical manufacturers spend approximately twice as much on marketing as they do on research and development. Pharmaceutical sponsors and manufacturers' provision of free drug samples has been criticized because of the perceived possibility that providers will be more likely to prescribe those drugs, which are often more expensive for the patient than what the provider might have otherwise prescribed.[32] Since passage of the PPACA in 2010, the FDA has regulated drug sample reporting.[33] Similarly, the Pharmaceutical Research and Manufacturers of America, representing research-based pharmaceutical companies, has developed promotional drug materials and education strategies that are consistent with FDA requirements governing drug-related communications.[34]

SUMMARY

Among its many duties, the FDA serves to protect the safety and health of consumers. The administration's primary drug review center, the CDER, processes investigational and NDAs via a 3-phase clinical trial period, followed by continued drug surveillance after release. New drugs are reviewed via standard or expedited reviews, with approval goals of 10 months and 6 months, respectively. The FDA has responded to criticism from government and nongovernment agencies regarding its regulatory practices and biases in the drug approval process. Passage of recent Acts, including the FDASIA, reflects the FDA's efforts toward ensuring greater agency transparency, increased vigilance during the drug development and approval process, and fiscal responsibility.

REFERENCES

1. Collins S, Rasmussen P, Doty M, et al. The rise in health care coverage and affordability since health reform took effect. New York: Commonwealth Fund; 2015. Available at: http://www.commonwealthfund.org/publications/issue-briefs/2015/jan/biennial-health-insurance-survey. Accessed July 8, 2015.
2. Schumock GT, Li EC, Suda KJ, et al. National trends in prescription drug expenditures and projections for 2015. Am J Health Syst Pharm 2015;72(9):717–36.

3. Ciociola AA, Cohen LB, Kulkarni P, et al. How drugs are developed and approved by the FDA: current process and future directions. Am J Gastroenterol 2014; 109(5):620–3.
4. Mullin R. Cost to develop new pharmaceutical drug now exceeds $2.5B. Available at: http://www.scientificamerican.com/article/cost-to-develop-new-pharmaceutical-drug-now-exceeds-2-5b/. Accessed August 6, 2015.
5. Mullard A. 2011 FDA Drug Approvals. Nat Rev Drug Discov 2012;11(2):91–4.
6. FDA Strategic Priorities 2014–2018. US Food and Drug Administration. Available at: http://www.fda.gov/downloads/AboutFDA/ReportsManualsForms/Reports/UCM416602.pdf. Accessed June 10, 2015.
7. Lee K, Bacchetti P, Sim I. Publication of clinical trials supporting successful new drug applications: a literature analysis. PLoS Med 2008;5(9):e191.
8. Porta M. A dictionary of epidemiology. 5th edition. New York: Oxford University Press; 2014.
9. Title 21, Part 201–Labeling. Code of federal regulations. Available at: www.accessdata.fda.gov/scripts/cdrh/cfdocs/cfcfr/cfrsearch.cfm?fr=201.56. Accessed July 21, 2015.
10. Kremzner M, Osborne S. An introduction to the improved FDA prescription drug labeling. US Food and Drug Administration. Available at: http://www.fda.gov/downloads/Training/ForHealthProfessionals/UCM090796.pdf. Accessed August 1, 2015.
11. Murphy S, Roberts R. 'Black box' 101: how the Food and Drug Administration evaluates, communicates, and manages drug benefit/risk. J Allergy Clin Immunol 2006;117(1):34–9.
12. Development & Approval Process (Drugs). US Food and Drug Administration. Available at: http://www.fda.gov/Drugs/DevelopmentApprovalProcess/. Accessed July 11, 2015.
13. Office of Pharmaceutical Quality. US Food and Drug Administration. Available at: http://www.fda.gov/AboutFDA/CentersOffices/OfficeofMedicalProductsandTobacco/CDER/ucm418347.htm. Accessed July 10, 2015.
14. Title 21, part 314–Applications for FDA Approval to Market a New Drug. Code of Federal Regulations. Available at: http://www.accessdata.fda.gov/scripts/cdrh/cfdocs/cfcfr/CFRsearch.cfm?CFRPart=314. Accessed July 21, 2015.
15. O'Connor AB. Building comparative efficacy and tolerability into the FDA approval process. JAMA 2010;303(10):979–80.
16. Center For Drug Evaluation and Research History–A Brief History of the Center for Drug Evaluation and Research–Slide Show. US Food and Drug Administration. Available at: http://www.fda.gov/AboutFDA/WhatWeDo/History/FOrgsHistory/CDER/ucm325199.htm. Accessed August 1, 2015.
17. Barley SR. Corporations, democracy, and the public good. J Manag Inq 2007; 16(3):201–15.
18. FDAReview.org, a project of the independent institute. FDAReview.org. Available at: http://fdareview.org/. Accessed July 27, 2015.
19. Kramer DB, Kesselheim AS. User fees and beyond–the FDA safety and innovation act of 2012. N Engl J Med 2012;367(14):1277–9.
20. Thaul S. How FDA approves drugs and regulates their safety and effectiveness. Washington, DC: Congressional Research Services; 2012. Available at: https://fas.org/sgp/crs/misc/R41983.pdf. Accessed May 10, 2015.
21. Jackson J. FDAMA 1997 Section 114: another look. Value Health 2009;12(2):191–2.
22. Stoltzfus T. An affordable care act at year 5: key issues for improvement. JAMA 2015;313(17):1709–10.

23. Thaul S, Bagalman E, Corby-Edwards A, et al. The Food and Drug Administration Safety and Innovation Act. 2012.
24. Information for Consumers (Drugs). The FDA's drug review process: ensuring drugs are safe and effective. US Food and Drug Administration. Available at: http://www.fda.gov/Drugs/ResourcesForYou/Consumers/ucm143534.htm. Accessed June 10, 2015.
25. Lee JY, Garnett CE, Gobburu JVS, et al. Impact of pharmacometric analyses on new drug approval and labeling decisions. Clin Pharmacokinet 2011;50(10): 627–35.
26. Thaul S. FDA fast track and priority review programs. Washington, DC: Congressional Research Service; 2008. Available at: http://nationalaglawcenter.org/wp-content/uploads/assets/crs/RS22814.pdf. Accessed June 1, 2011.
27. Suvarna V. Phase IV of drug development. Perspect Clin Res 2010;2:57–60.
28. Qato DM, Alexander CG. Improving the Food and Drug Administration's mandate to ensure postmarketing drug safety. JAMA 2011;306(14):1595–6.
29. Guidance for Industry: Format and Content of Proposed Risk Evaluation and Mitigation Strategies. FDA. Available at: http://www.fda.gov/downloads/drugs/guidancecomplianceregulatoryinformation/guidances/UCM184128.pdf. Accessed May 1, 2015.
30. Roberts SA, Allen JD, Sigal EV. Despite criticism of the FDA review process, new cancer drugs reach patients sooner in the United States than in Europe. Health Aff 2011;30(7):1375–81.
31. Gagnon M-A, Lexchin J. The cost of pushing pills: a new estimate of pharmaceutical promotion expenditures in the United States. PLoS Med 2008;5(1):e1.
32. Hurley MP, Stafford RS, Lane AT. Characterizing the relationship between free drug samples and prescription patterns for acne Vulgaris and Rosacea. JAMA Dermatology 2014;150(5):487.
33. Affordable Care Act Section 6004. 2010. Available at: www.fda.gov/drugs/guidance/complianceregulatoryinformation/ucm297609.htm. Accessed August 1, 2015.
34. Code on Interactions with Healthcare Professionals. Pharmaceutical research and manufacturers of America. Available at: http://www.phrma.org/sites/default/files/pdf/phrma_marketing_code_2008-1.pdf. Accessed August 1, 2015.

Heart Failure

Overcoming the Physiologic Dilemma Through Evidence-Based Practice

Sheila Melander, PhD, ACNP-BC, FCCM, FAANP[a],*,
Stephen Miller, ANP, MSN, ACNP-BC[b]

KEYWORDS

- Heart failure • Evidence-based practice • Reduced ejection fraction
- Preserved ejection fraction • Treatment

KEY POINTS

- Heart failure occurs with a decline in myocardial performance leading to pulmonary and systemic congestion.
- The pathophysiologic derangement of systolic and diastolic heart failure and right heart failure differ dramatically, necessitating a focused, evidenced-based treatment regimen.
- Disease classification and treatment guidelines from the American Heart Association and the American College of Cardiology play a key role in the treatment paradigm.
- Nonpharmacologic interventions (eg, fluid and sodium restriction, daily weights, obesity management, hypertension management, exercise, routine vaccines, and tobacco cessation) are the foundation of treatment.
- There is a robust body of evidence to prove that pharmacologic interventions reduce morbidity and mortality of heart failure.

Cardiovascular disease remains the leading global cause of death, with 17.3 million deaths per year. This astounding statistic is expected to increase to 23.6 million by 2030. Within that label the prevalence of heart failure (HF) remains a major public health problem of more than 5.8 million in the United States and more than 23 million worldwide.[1] In 2011, 1 in 9 death certificates in the United States mentioned HF. The number of any-mention deaths attributable to HF was approximately as high in 1995 as it was in 2011, and hospital discharges for HF remained stable from 2000 to 2010.[2] Total costs for HF were estimated to be $30.7 billion in 2012. Of this total, 68% was attributable to direct medical costs. Projections show that by 2030, the total cost of HF will increase almost 127% to $69.7 billion from 2012.[2]

Disclosures: Speaker agreement with Novartis Pharmaceutical.
[a] Norton's Healthcare System, University of Kentucky, 3682 Briarcliff Trace, Owensboro, KY 42303, USA; [b] Tennova Turkey Creek Medical Center, 10810 Parkside Drive, Knoxville, TN 37934, USA
* Corresponding author.
E-mail address: sheila.melander@uky.edu

Nurs Clin N Am 51 (2016) 13–27
http://dx.doi.org/10.1016/j.cnur.2015.11.004
0029-6465/16/$ – see front matter © 2016 Elsevier Inc. All rights reserved.

Treatment paradigms revolve around primary and secondary prevention models. Age, coronary artery disease, valvular disease, and poorly controlled hypertension are identified as major contributing factors in the development of HF. Hypertension remains the leading contributor to HF, with 75% of HF cases having antecedent hypertension.[2] Our health care system is burdened by escalating medical costs, and the need for evidence-based best practices to contain this increasing burden is great. As survival rates among patients with cardiovascular disease and, specifically, HF continue to increase, strategies to improve our utilization of evidence-based therapies and interventions to prevent and manage HF are required.

PATHOPHYSIOLOGY

Hypertension, ischemic coronary disease, idiopathic myopathies, and valvular disorders are among the initial causes leading to HF. Heart failure is characterized by a decline in myocardial performance which leads to a decrease in exercise tolerance and ultimately pulmonary and systemic congestion. Although cardiac remodeling occurs at the organ, cellular, and molecular levels and is compensatory, it becomes a progressive and lethal process. This derangement further decreases myocardial function and increases arrhythmia potential, which are the major causes of morbidity and mortality in patients with HF.[3] Patients with HF experience congestive symptoms and vacillate between states of compensation and decompensation. HF is classified as congestive HF with reduced ejection fraction (HFrEF) and congestive HF with preserved ejection fraction (HFpEF). The cause of each differs substantially.

Heart Failure with Reduced Ejection Fraction

HF with reduced ejection fraction, also known as systolic HF, results from the destructive outcomes of ischemic processes, such as coronary artery disease. Nonischemic cardiomyopathy represents another type of HFrEF with genetic, viral, chemotherapeutic, valvular, and alcoholic causes. In both ischemic and nonischemic cases, myocardial injury and maladaptive myocyte compensation lead to remodeling of the left ventricle and a cascade of neurohormonal responses (eg, sympathetic stimulation, renin-angiotensin-aldosterone, endothelin, epinephrine, growth hormone, cortisol, tumor necrosis factor, prostaglandins, substance P, adrenomedullin, and natriuretic peptides) that further impact the failing left ventricle.[4,5] Sympathetic nervous system activation provides inotropic drive for the failing heart, resulting in increased stroke volume and peripheral vasoconstriction in a compensatory attempt to maintain mean arterial perfusion pressure. The renin-angiotensin aldosterone system (RAAS) is a compensatory mechanism to maintain homeostatic control of mean arterial pressure, tissue perfusion, and extracellular volume. The role of endogenous natriuretic peptides in protecting against sodium and volume overload is well recognized, and this family of peptides is thought to have a range of other beneficial cardiac, vascular, and renal actions.[6] Current research reveals the role tissue neutral endopeptidase (NEP) plays in HF treatment by cleaving and inactivating the natriuretic peptides. NEP inhibition has been shown to increase endogenous atrial natriuretic peptide and B-type natriuretic peptide (BNP) levels in association with beneficial hemodynamic and renal effects in HF.[7] Neurohormonal activation has net effects that include vasoconstriction, volume expansion, tachycardia, and inotropic stimulation.[8] These compensatory mechanisms continue cycling as the pathophysiologic response to the failing pump. The optimal myocardial threshold is surpassed, and systolic dysfunction results in cardiac remodeling that increases preload and afterload, thus, increasing left ventricle size and wall stress. Geometric changes cause electrophysiologic and structural abnormalities (eg, mitral regurgitation) and further degrade the myocardial efficiency and increase wall stress.[9] Manifestations of the failing left ventricle include fatigue, dyspnea (on exertion or progressively at rest), orthopnea, paroxysmal nocturnal dyspnea, nocturia, mental status changes, and abdominal pain.[10]

Pharmacologic and nonpharmacologic therapies are initiated to address these symptoms and prevent further progression.

Heart Failure with Preserved Ejection Fraction

Causes of HF with preserved ejection fraction (HFpEF) include hypertension (and a suspected hypertensive cause) and diabetes with hypertension as an independent predictor of HFpEF in hospitalized patients.[11,12] The term *diastolic HF* is used interchangeably with HFpEF. Underlying diastolic function abnormalities are the hallmarks of HF with preserved ejection fraction.[13,14] The presence of abnormal active relaxation and increased passive stiffness results in increased diastolic pressures and signs and symptoms of HF in this group of patients.[15,16] These patients often have cardiogenic pulmonary edema as a result of sodium retention and central blood volume expansion.[17] Elevated diastolic filling pressures are a result of increased passive chamber stiffness. Consequently, high filling pressures degrade lung compliance and cause an increase in the work of breathing and dyspnea.[15] The dilemma of a noncompliant stiff ventricle is a reduction in efficiency and subsequent mismatch between supply and demand (eg, Frank-Starling mechanism).[18] When challenged during exertion, the noncompliant stiff ventricle has high filling pressures and cannot fill efficiently. The left ventricle cannot meet physiologic demands and increased cardiac output, which further exacerbates symptoms of dyspnea.[15] A thorough understanding of the pathophysiology of diastolic HF is important in applying pharmacologic intervention to this group of patients. The current body of evidence supports the use of angiotensin-converting enzyme inhibitors (ACE-Is), alpha receptor blockers, beta-blockers, and calcium channel blockers in the treatment of this condition.

Right Heart Failure

The leading cause of right HF is pulmonary artery hypertension (PAH) secondary to pulmonary vasculopathy. Anatomically, the right ventricle (RV) is thinner than the left ventricle as a result of reduced afterload in the pulmonary vasculature. In PAH, pulmonary pressures escalate providing vascular resistance on the RV. Sustained pressure overload causes the RV to lose contractile force and to increase thickness of the wall. This increased thickness is referred to as RV hypertrophy (RVH). Functional, structural, and numerical changes in cardiomyocytes cause a vicious cycle of further compromised contractility and dilatation. Autocrine, paracrine, and neuroendocrine signaling pathways are an attempt by the body to compensate for the decline in contractility and progress to further deterioration. Therapies aimed at treating right HF are currently evolving and focusing on the transition from compensated RVH to maladaptive remodeling and dilatation.[19,20]

THE CHRONIC TO ACUTE CONTINUUM

Patients with HF fluctuate on a continuum of the chronic disease state from compensated to acute decompensation. The American College of Cardiology Foundation (ACCF) in conjunction with the American Heart Association (AHA) classifies specific stages that define where patients are on the continuum of chronicity. HF can be classified in 2 different manners as highlighted in **Table 1**. This 4-staged classification starts with identification of patients at risk for the development of HF and ends with refractory HF. The New York Heart Association (NYHA) classifies HF according to functional status. Patients with HF present with a wide variety of signs and symptoms, which can range from dyspnea and symptoms of fluid overload to others who have no symptoms of congestion but have signs of low cardiac output, such as cachexia, fatigue, and renal hypoperfusion. The NYHA classification is used to assess the functional limitations and has been shown to correlate with prognosis.

Both are used in the diagnosis and management of patients with HF. Once patients are identified in a particular stage or class, as the disease progresses or advances, so does the stage or classification. Interventions are identified for each stage or classification with the purpose of modifying risk factors, reducing morbidity and mortality rates, as well as the treatment of structural heart disease. These stages and classifications can be used in conjunction to assist in identification of stages, diagnosis, and treatment strategies (see **Table 1**).[23]

EVIDENCE-BASED MANAGEMENT

Once patients are diagnosed with HF, depending on the stage or classification, both nonpharmacologic and pharmacologic measures may be used.

Table 1
Comparison of ACCF/AHA stages of HF and NYHA functional classifications

ACCF/AHA Stages of HF[21]		NYHA Functional Classification[22]
A At high risk for HF but without structural heart disease or symptoms of HF	None	—
B Structural heart disease but without signs or symptoms of HF	I	There is no limitation of physical activity. Ordinary physical activity does not cause symptoms of HF.
C Structural heart disease with prior or current symptoms of HF	I	There is no limitation of physical activity. Ordinary physical activity does not cause symptoms of HF.
	II	There is slight limitation of physical activity. Patients are comfortable at rest, but ordinary physical activity results in symptoms of HF.
	III	There is marked limitation of physical activity. Patients are comfortable at rest, but less than ordinary activity causes symptoms of HF.
	IV	Patients are unable to carry on any physical activity without symptoms of HF, or there are symptoms of HF at rest.
D Refractory HF requiring specialized interventions	IV	Patients are unable to carry on any physical activity without symptoms of HF, or there are symptoms of HF at rest.

Abbreviation: NYHA, New York Heart Association.

Data from Hunt SA, Baker DW, Chin MH, et al. ACC/AHA guidelines for the evaluation and management of chronic heart failure in the adult: executive summary a report of the American College of Cardiology/American Heart Association Task Force on Practice Guidelines (committee to revise the 1995 guidelines for the evaluation and management of heart failure): developed in collaboration with the International Society for Heart and Lung Transplantation; endorsed by the Heart Failure Society of America. Circulation 2001;104:2996–3007; and Farrell MH, Foody JM, Krumholz HM. Beta-blockers in heart failure: clinical applications. JAMA 2002;287(7):890–7.

NONPHARMACOLOGIC
Fluid and Sodium Restrictions

Patients diagnosed with HF are typically asked to implement a sodium- and fluid-restricted diet. Usually patients are limited to 2 g/d of sodium and a total of 2 L of fluid per day. These measures will decrease the vascular congestion as well as decrease the need for diuretic therapy. Fluid restrictions might be more stringent in acute exacerbations of HF. Patients are asked to monitor their daily weight and may have protocols individually designed around particular weight variations, which might include increased diuretic therapy.

Management of Hypertension

Hypertension has been identified as a major risk factor in the development of HF. This risk encompasses all ages and sexes. Long-term treatment of hypertension, resulting in control of hypertension, has been shown to reduce the risk of HF by 50%. Assuring that patients understand the important consequences of uncontrolled hypertension must be a priority. Treatment of hypertension has been especially beneficial in the elderly population. An initial high blood pressure reading and tendencies toward high blood pressure should be addressed immediately. Sodium- and fluid-restricted diets and stress reduction therapy and/or biofeedback are options to address this finding nonpharmacologically. Causes such as renal artery stenosis or other physiologic processes contributing to the hypertension should be explored. In cases whereby nonpharmacologic measures are unsuccessful, choices for antihypertensive therapy should be discussed with the provider and considered with regard to comorbidities, such as diabetes, thyroid disease, or coronary artery disease. Diuretic therapy as well as ACE-Is, angiotensin receptor blockers (ARBs), and beta-blocker therapy are potentially viable options but should be individualized with optimal[24,25] outcomes for all comorbidities.[26,27]

Obesity

Obesity has been linked to an increase in HF. Risk factors associated with obesity include diabetes, sleep apnea, and metabolic syndrome. Sleep disorders, such as sleep apnea, are common in patients with HF. A study of patients diagnosed with HF showed that 61% had either obstructive or central sleep apnea. It is important to ask if your patients snore or if their significant other has noted snoring or apneic periods during sleep. Patients may also complain of daytime somnolence and extreme fatigue. Sleep studies are recommended if patients exhibit these symptoms, and treatment is usually nocturnal continuous positive airway pressure (C-PAP). Studies have shown the use of C-PAP improved oxygenation, increased left ventricular ejection fraction (LVEF), and distance able to walk in 6 minutes. Research showed that the benefits persisted for up to 2 years.[28–30]

Tobacco and Alcohol Use

Tobacco use has been strongly associated with HF. Patients who smoke should be counseled and smoking cessation efforts advised and established. Patients should discuss options with their providers to achieve optimal outcomes for cessation.[31,32] Alcohol has been identified with the development of HF, although there is variance around the amount consumed and the likelihood of HF. There are some sex differences around consumption; however, consensus exists that heavy use of alcohol repeatedly has been associated with increased risks for the development of HF. Patients should be advised as to the level of their consumption and the risks associated for the development of HF.[33–35]

Exercise

Regular physical exercise is safe and has been shown to have many benefits for patients with HF. In patients with HF, cardiac rehabilitation involving increased exercise or duration improves functional capacity, has decreased mortality rates, and has resulted in reduction in the number of hospitalizations.[21,36]

In addition to the nonpharmacologic therapies discussed earlier, electrophysiologic therapies (such as cardiac resynchronization or defibrillator implantation) and/or surgical interventions (including implantation of left ventricular assist devices or cardiac transplantation) may be used.

Routine Vaccinations

Pneumococcal vaccine and annual influenza vaccination are recommended in all patients diagnosed with HF unless contraindicated. Regularly scheduled follow-up visits and the importance of these visits need to be emphasized and understood by patients.

PHARMACOLOGIC MANAGEMENT
Diuretic Therapy

Diuretic therapy is the standard treatment of patients with HF and has been shown to improve symptoms and exercise tolerance.[22] Loop, thiazide, and potassium-sparing diuretics all may be considered. Thiazide diuretics are used in hypertensive patients that have mild fluid retention and seem to have better antihypertensive effects. The goal of diuretic therapy is to decrease fluid accumulation or retention. Diuretic therapy is usually combined with a decrease in fluid intake and sodium restriction. Diuretics are usually prescribed based on a dosing schedule, which often needs adjustment once patients return home. Patients can become resistant or unresponsive to high doses of diuretics, especially if they consume large amounts of sodium or are taking other medications that may block the effects of the diuretic. Some drugs that have the potential to do this include nonsteroidal antiinflammatory drugs. Renal impairment can also alter the efficacy of diuretics in some patients. Potassium-sparing medications are helpful in the management of patients with HF who may have electrolyte disturbances or other cardiac comorbidities.[37–39] **Table 2** shows commonly used oral diuretics in the treatment of HF.

Aldosterone Antagonist

Aldosterone inhibitors prevent sodium and water retention as well as myocardial fibrosis. Use of these drugs requires frequent monitoring of potassium levels and renal function and should be avoided in patients with creatinine levels greater than 2.5 mg/dL. Studies have shown a 30% reduction in mortality rates and hospitalizations when spironolactone is added to standardized therapy for patients with HF with NYHA class III or IV. A 15% reduction of mortality and hospitalization was reported in patients with NYHA class II to IV with LVEF less than 40% after a myocardial infarction who were treated with eplerenone. Gynecomastia has been noted in 8% of patients who have taken spironolactone, but this has not been reported with the use of eplerenone. The dosing of spironolactone can be found in the **Table 2**. Eplerenone should be started at 25 mg daily with a maximum dose of 50 mg.[40,41]

Table 2
Diuretics commonly used in the treatment of HF

Drug	Initial Daily Dose	Maximum Daily Dose
Loop diuretics		
Bumetanide	0.5–1.0 mg once or twice	10 mg
Furosemide	20–40 mg once or twice	600 mg
Torsemide	10–20 mg once	200 mg
Thiazide diuretics		
Hydrochlorothiazide	25 mg once or twice	200 mg
Chlorothiazide	250–500 mg once or twice	1000 mg
Chlorthalidone	12.5–25.0 mg once	100 mg
Indapamide	2.5 mg once	5 mg
Metolazone	2.5 mg once	20 mg
Potassium-sparing diuretics		
Spironolactone	12.5–25.0 mg once	50 mg
Triamterene	50–75 mg twice	200 mg

Angiotensin-Converting Enzyme Inhibitors

ACE-Is prevent the conversion of angiotensin-1 to angiotensin II. Angiotensin II is a strong vasoconstrictor and also promotes the production of aldosterone. Aldosterone promotes sodium and water retention in the body. By inhibiting the production of angiotensin II, ACE-Is promote vasodilatation and the prevention of fluid volume increases. All patients with left ventricular systolic dysfunction should be treated with an ACE-I unless they have a contraindication or sensitivity/intolerance to the drug. ACE-Is have been shown to reduce mortality and hospitalizations seen in patients with HF that also have known reduced LVEF. ACE-Is should be prescribed with caution to those with low systemic blood pressure (systolic <80), renal artery stenosis, elevated serum creatinine levels (>5.0 mEq/L), high serum creatinine (>3 mg/dL), or previous angioedema with use. ACE-I therapy should be started at low doses and titrated slowly as needed and as tolerated. Renal function as well as potassium levels should be assessed within 1 to 2 weeks of initiation of therapy and after dose alterations. Doses should be prescribed that have been shown to reduce the risks of cardiovascular events in clinical trials. If patients cannot tolerate the targeted dose, intermediate doses should be used as there have been minimal differences noted in the efficacy between low and high doses. Sudden withdrawal of ACE-Is should be avoided as they can cause clinical deterioration and decreases in LVEF. Up to 20% of patients may complain of an ACE-induced cough. If this interferes with activities of daily living or interrupts sleep, ARBs therapy can be very helpful. ACE-I therapy should be used in combination with beta-blockers unless contraindicated, and either therapy can be initiated first.[42,43] **Table 3** presents commonly used ACE-Is with suggested dosing.

Angiotensin Receptor Blockers

ACE-Is remain the first line of therapy, but ARBs are now considered an alternative. ARBs have many of the same considerations as ACE-I use and should be considered before initiation of therapy. ARBs are recommended as alternate therapy in patients who do not tolerate ACE-Is because of cough or angioedema.[44,45] **Table 4** shows commonly used angiotensin receptor blocking agents with recommended dosing.

Table 3 ACE-I		
Drug	**Target Dose**	**Frequency**
Enalapril	20 mg	bid
Lisinopril	40 mg	qd
Captopril	50 mg	tid
Ramipril	5 mg	bid
Benazepril	20 mg	qd
Quinapril	20 mg	bid

Beta-Blocker Therapy

Stable patients with HF who have reduced LVEF are recommended to receive beta-blocker therapy unless contraindicated. Patients with severe lung disease, bronchospasm, bradycardia, or hypotension may not tolerate therapy. It is recommended that therapy begin before discharged from the hospital or on an outpatient basis started at low doses and titrated to the desired dose. Beta-blockers are given in combination with an ACE-I for optimal effect on increasing LVEF. Beta-blockers as a class have been proven to reduce morbidity and mortality rates. Carvedilol is the only agent approved by the Food and Drug Administration for treatment of patients with HF. Benefits were noted for patients with or without coronary artery disease, diabetes, as well as in women and African Americans.

Beta-blocker therapy can produce different types of adverse effects. Fluid retention, worsening HF, bradycardia or heart block, and hypotension have been noted. Fatigue is another frequent complaint, which can be multifactorial and the most difficult to address. As with all other therapy, close monitoring and frequent visits will help guide for optimal outcomes.[46,47] See **Table 5** for initial and targeting dosing.

Digoxin

Digoxin overall increases the efficiency of the heart's ability to contract, increasing the strength of contraction and is also effective in controlling the rate and rhythm. Digoxin increases the force of contractions by inhibiting an enzyme (adenosinetriphosphatase), which controls movement of calcium, sodium, and potassium within the heart muscle. Digoxin also slows conduction between the atrium and the ventricles and is helpful in decreasing heart rates and in the management of some arrhythmias. Several trials have shown that use of digoxin for 1 to 3 months can improve symptoms, heart rate, and exercise tolerance for patients with HF. In a long-term trial, patients with NYHA class II or III, treatment of 2 to 5 years had no effect on mortality rates but

Table 4 ARB dosing		
Agent	**Initial Dose (mg)**	**Maximum Dose (mg)**
Drug	**Dose**	**Frequency**
Valsartan	80	320
Candesartan	4	32
Losartan	25	100
Irbesartan	75	300
Telmisartan	40	80

Table 5
Beta-blocker dosing

Beta-Blocker	Initial Dosage	Maximal Target Dosage
Carvedilol	3.125 mg bid	50 mg bid if >75 kg 25 mg bid if <75 kg
Sustained-release metoprolol succinate	12.5 mg qd	200 mg qd
Bisoprolol	2.5 mg qd	10 mg qd

had a modest effect on reducing the combined risk of hospitalization and death. Digoxin may be prescribed for patients with left ventricular systolic dysfunction who remain symptomatic while receiving medical therapy, particularly those who also have atrial fibrillation. Digoxin is usually started at a low dosage of 0.125 mg daily. The maximum dosage is 0.25 mg daily, and guidelines recommend reduced dosages for women, patients with renal dysfunction, and those on amiodarone.[48,49]

Hydralazine and Nitrates

The combination of hydralazine and nitrates, such as isosorbide, is recommended for African Americans with NYHA class III to IV HF with reduced LVEF who remain symptomatic with the combined use of ACE-Is, beta-blockers, and aldosterone antagonists. Combined therapy for hydralazine and nitrates is also suggested if patients are intolerant to ACE-Is or ARB therapy. If fixed dosing is available, the initial dosage should be 37.5 mg hydralazine hydrochloride and 20 mg isosorbide dinitrate 3 times daily. The dosage can be increased to 2 tablets 3 times daily if needed. Adherence to this combination has generally been poor because of the number of tablets and frequency required. Frequent adverse effects include headache, dizziness, and gastrointestinal complaints.

Hydralazine and nitrates may be added to ACE-Is and beta-blockers when additional afterload reduction is needed or if pulmonary hypertension is noted.[50]

INTRAVENOUS INOTROPES AND VASODILATORS
Dobutamine

Dobutamine is a beta-receptor agonist, which enhances contractility by directly stimulating the beta-1 receptors. For patients with acute hypotensive HF or shock, the use of dobutamine may be helpful when guided by hemodynamic monitoring. The dose is usually titrated to the lowest dose to achieve the hemodynamic goals. Long-term use of infusions of dobutamine can increase mortality, especially because of its arrhythmogenic effects, and are not recommended for routine management of HF. Chronic dobutamine infusions are reserved for palliative use for patients who already have implantable cardioverter-defibrillators (ICDs) and are waiting for heart transplantation. Dobutamine is started generally at 2 mg/kg/min and can be titrated to 20 mg/kg/min.[51]

Milrinone

Milrinone is an inotrope and also a vasodilator. Milrinone is helpful for patients on chronic oral beta-blocker therapy who develop HF. It is also used in patients with low-output HF and pulmonary hypertension because it is a potent pulmonary vasodilator. The Outcomes of a Prospective Trail of Intravenous Milrinone for Exacerbations of Chronis Heart Failure involved routine intravenous (IV) infusions of milrinone for those with decompensated HF. The study failed to show clinical benefit and was associated with increased arrhythmias and hypotension. Thus, milrinone currently is not recommended for routine management of HF.[52]

ANTICOAGULATION

Patients who have been diagnosed with HF are at higher risks for the development of atrial fibrillation and subsequent clot formation. Progression of atrial fibrillation goes from approximately 4% in NYHA class 1% to 40% in class VI. Patients who have been diagnosed with HF and also have paroxysmal atrial fibrillation require anticoagulation with agents such as warfarin, dabigatran, apixaban, or rivaroxaban. The medication is selected based on risk, cost, patient preference, and possible reaction with other prescribed medications. Patients on warfarin sodium (Coumadin) or warfarin will need to be monitored for therapeutic international normalized ratio levels.[53,54]

NEW AND EMERGING THERAPIES

New and emerging therapies for HF management are showing significant impact on cardiovascular outcomes and should be considered. The PARADIGM-HF (Prospective comparison of ARNI with ACEI to determine Impact of Global Mortality and Morbidity in HF) trial is a large randomized trial that evaluated secubitril/valsartan and is indicated to reduce the risk of cardiovascular death and hospitalization for HF in patients with chronic HF (CHF) (NYHA class II–IV) and reduced ejection fraction.[55] LCZ696 belongs to a new class of drugs, the angiotensin receptor neprilys inhibitors, which both block the RAAS and augment natriuretic peptides. Its mechanism of action occurs through angiotensin receptor-neprilysin inhibition. Additionally, Ivabrandine is a hyperpolarization-activated cyclic nucleotide-gated channel blocker that was evaluated in the SHIFT (Systolic Heart failure trial with the If inhibitor Ivabrandine) trial and is shown to reduce the risk of hospitalization and cardiovascular death in patients with chronic NYHA class II to IV CHF.[56]

DIFFERING VIEWS ON THE USE OF INTRAVENOUS NESIRITIDE (NATRECOR)

Nesiritide is a human recombinant form of BNP, which mimics the action of endogenous BNP. Natrecor or nesiritide has diuretic, natriuretic, vasodilatory, and smooth muscle actions. It has no proarrhythmic effects and has been given to patients in acute HF in the past but has been shown in the ASCEND-HF (Acute Study of Clinical Effectiveness of Nesiritide and Decompensated heart failure) trial as well as a 2013 multicenter study to have little or no effect on dyspnea and no significant effect on morbidity or readmission rates in addition to hypotensive events. Recommendations from both of these studies were that nesiritide not be used as routine outpatient, scheduled, or repetitive infusions. Additionally, it was not recommended for use in dyspnea or to increase diuresis. Subsequent data from the Acute Decompensated Heart Failure National Registry (ADHERE) show that nesiritide is devoid of proarrhythmic risks when compared with inotrope therapy and has confirmed the safety of nesiritide and nitrates over inotropes. Data from the ADHERE registry showed that it was an effective IV vasodilator, which was well tolerated, not requiring titration, and without tolerance issues. Data also showed that the dose needed to provide rapid reduced filling pressures and relief of symptoms could be an issue in the preservation of renal function, suggesting further study needed.[57–66]

PALLIATIVE CARE

Patients who have been diagnosed with end-stage HF fall into stage D of the ACC/AHA classification system and class III to IV of the NYHA functional classification system. Every attempt must be made to identify and reverse causes for worsening

HF, such as poor compliance, arrhythmias, valvular regurgitation, pulmonary embolism, renal dysfunction, or infection. Once all strategies have been exhausted, patients with end-stage HF need continuity of medical care between outpatient and inpatient settings.

Before patients become too debilitated to actively participate in their care decisions, it is of utmost importance for them to be well educated about options for the formulation and implementation of advance practice initiatives. It will be important to ask what role they want the palliative services or hospice care services to provide. It is also important to educate patients and families that patient needs may change dramatically and periodic reevaluations are necessary. Discussions need to include preference for resuscitation in the event of cardiopulmonary arrest, life-sustaining measures if any are desired, and the inactivation of the ICD at the end of life. It is also necessary to help all involved understand that aggressive or heroic measures, such as intubation or ICD implantation, in the final days of patients who are NYHA class IV will not result in clinical improvement or improved clinical outcomes and are not appropriate measures.[67]

As patients move toward end-stage failure, hospice may provide options that alleviate pain and suffering, depression, fear, and insomnia. Other treatments may include psychological support, increased use of opiates, frequent or continuous use of IV diuretics, positive inotropic agents, oxygen, anxiolytics, and sleeping medications. In the final days, it may become very difficult for the patients, providers, and family members to discern or define the point in time when the patients' care changes from improving survival to improving quality of life and, thus, allowing for a dignified and peaceful death.

SUMMARY

There are few protocol-driven therapies, which were again stressed in the recent 2013 ACCF/AHA guidelines for the management of patients with HF.[23]

1. Diuretics are needed in most patients to manage fluid retention.
2. All patients with HF should receive an ACE-I and a beta-blocker unless contraindicated.
3. Use of aldosterone antagonists improve survival and prevent hospitalizations.
4. Digoxin is reserved for patients with signs and symptoms of HF.
5. Hydralazine plus a nitrate may be added to ACE-Is and a beta-blocker to provide additional symptomatic relief.

Treatment options for patients with HF have improved in recent years. Medication combinations along with improved device management have improved patient survival rates and improved quality of life for our HF patient population. It is important to note that most patients with HF are older than 65 years. Nearly half of the older patients with HF have HF with preserved LVEF, and nearly half with HF with reduced LVEF are octogenarians. Because patients with HF with multiple comorbidities and with any physical or cognitive impairments are often excluded from trials or studies, there is little evidence to truly guide therapy for most of the older patients with HF.[68] Health care providers must always remember that our older patients with HF with multiple comorbidities and polypharmacy are at great risks for adverse effects and drug-to-drug interactions. These factors are all strong reasons for individualized therapy, which includes active input from patients and families. Customized therapy in conjunction with provider involvement at all points of patient care can help us to continue to improve HF outcomes.

REFERENCES

1. Roger VL. Epidemiology of heart failure. Circ Res 2013;113(6):646–59.
2. Mozaffarian D, Benjamin EJ, Go AS, et al, on behalf of the American Heart Association Statistics Committee and Stroke Statistics Subcommittee. Heart disease and stroke statistics—2015 update: a report from the American Heart Association. Circulation 2015;131:e29–322.
3. Wilson R, Chen X, Houser S. Congestive heart failure: cellular and molecular abnormalities in failing cardiac myocytes. 3rd edition. Philadelphia: Lippencott Williams; 2007. p. 15–25.
4. McMurray J. Systolic heart failure. N Engl J Med 2010;362:228–38.
5. Gomberg-Maitland M, Baran DA, Fuster V. Treatment of congestive heart failure: guidelines for the primary care physician and the heart failure specialist. Arch Intern Med 2001;161(3):342–52.
6. McMurray JJV, Packer M, Desai AS, et al, on behalf of the PARADIGM-HF Committees Investigators. Baseline characteristics and treatment of patients in Prospective comparison of ARNI with ACEI to Determine Impact on Global Mortality and morbidity in Heart Failure trial (PARADIGM-HF). Eur J Heart Fail 2014;16:817–25.
7. Rademaker M, Charles C, Espiner E, et al. Combined neutral endopeptidase and angiotensin-converting enzyme inhibition in heart failure: role of natriuretic peptides and angiotensin II. J Cardiovasc Pharmacol 1998;131:116–25.
8. Braunwald E, Colucci W, Grossman W. Clinical aspects of heart failure: high output heart failure: pulmonary edema. In: Braunwald E, editor. Heart disease: a textbook of cardiovascular medicine. 9th edition. Philadelphia: WB Saunders Co; 1997. p. 445–56.
9. Packer M, Cohn J. Consensus recommendations for the management of chronic heart failure. Am J Cardiol 1999;83(2A):831A–8A.
10. Irani SR. Psychological heart disease? Arch Intern Med 2001;161(3):485–6.
11. Hogg K, Swedberg K, McMurray J. Heart failure with preserved left ventricular systolic function: epidemiology, clinical characteristics, and prognosis. J Am Coll Cardiol 2004;43(3):317–27.
12. Vasan RS, Levy D. The role of hypertension in the pathogenesis of heart failure. A clinical mechanistic overview. Arch Intern Med 1996;156:1789–96, 41.
13. Sanjay K, Gandhi M, John C, et al. The pathogenesis of acute pulmonary edema associated with hypertension. N Engl J Med 2001;344:17–22.
14. Redfield MM, Jacobsen SJ, Burnett JC Jr, et al. Burden of systolic and diastolic ventricular dysfunction in the community: appreciating the scope of the heart failure epidemic. JAMA 2003;289(2):194–202.
15. Zile MR, Baicu CF, Gaasch WH. Diastolic heart failure: abnormalities in active relaxation and passive stiffness of the left ventricle. N Engl J Med 2004;350:1953–9.
16. Vasan R, Levy D. Defining diastolic heart failure: a call for standardized diagnostic criteria. Circulation 2000;101:2118–21.
17. Chen H, Lainchbury J, Senni M, et al. Diastolic heart failure in the community: clinical profile, natural history, therapy, and impact of proposed diagnostic criteria. J Card Fail 2002;8:279–87.
18. Kitzman DW, Higginbotham MB, Cobb FR, et al. Exercise intolerance in patients with heart failure and preserved left ventricular systolic function: failure of the Frank-Starling mechanism. J Am Coll Cardiol 1991;17:1065–72.

19. Little WC, Kitzman DW, Cheng CP. Diastolic dysfunction as a cause of exercise intolerance. Heart Fail Rev 2000;5:301–6.
20. Bogaard HJ, Abe K, Vonk Noordegraaf A, et al. The right ventricle under pressure: cellular and molecular mechanisms of right-heart failure in pulmonary hypertension. Chest 2009;135(3):794–804.
21. Austin J, Williams R, Ross L, et al. Randomised controlled trial of cardiac rehabilitation in elderly patients with heart failure. Eur J Heart Fail 2005;7:411–7.
22. Horsley L. ACC and AHA update on chronic heart failure guidelines. Am Fam Physician 2010;81(5):654–65.
23. Yancy C, Jessup M, Butler J, et al. 2013 ACCF/AHA guideline for the management of heart failure: a report of the American College of Cardiology Foundation/American Heart Association Task Force on Practice Guidelines. Circulation 2013;128(16): 1810–52.
24. Beckett NS, Peters R, Fletcher AE, et al. Treatment of hypertension in patients 80 years of age or older. N Engl J Med 2008;358:1887–98, 312.
25. Sciarretta S, Palano F, Tocci G, et al. Antihypertensive treatment and development of heart failure in hypertension: a Bayesian network meta-analysis of studies in patients with hypertension and high cardiovascular risk. Arch Intern Med 2011; 171:384–94.
26. Staessen JA, Wang JG, Thijs L. Cardiovascular prevention and blood pressure reduction: a quantitative overview updated until 1 March 2003. J Hypertens 2003;21:1055–76.
27. Verdecchia P, Sleight P, Mancia G, et al. Effects of telmisartan, ramipril, and their combination on left ventricular hypertrophy in individuals at high vascular risk in the ongoing telmisartan alone and in combination with ramipril global end point trial and the telmisartan randomized assessment study in ACE intolerant subjects with cardiovascular disease. Circulation 2009;120:1380–9.
28. Bradley TD, Logan AG, Kimoff RJ, et al. Continuous positive air-way pressure for central sleep apnea and heart failure. N Engl J Med 2005;353:2025–33.
29. Kaneko Y, Floras JS, Usui K, et al. Cardiovascular effects of continuous positive airway pressure in patients with heart failure and obstructive sleep apnea. N Engl J Med 2003;348:1233–41.
30. Mansfield DR, Gollogly NC, Kaye DM, et al. Controlled trial of continuous positive airway pressure in obstructive sleep apnea and heart failure. Am J Respir Crit Care Med 2004;169:361–6.
31. Butler J, Kalogeropoulos A, Georgiopoulou V, et al. Incident heart failure prediction in the elderly: the Health ABC heart failure score. Circ Heart Fail 2008;1: 125–33.
32. Kalogeropoulos A, Georgiopoulou V, Kritchevsky SB, et al. Epidemiology of incident heart failure in a contemporary elderly cohort: the health, aging, and body composition study. Arch Intern Med 2009;169:708–15.
33. Wilhelmsen L, Rosengren A, Eriksson H, et al. Heart failure in the general population of men: morbidity, risk factors and prognosis. J Intern Med 2001;249: 253–61.
34. Abramson JL, Williams SA, Krumholz HM, et al. Moderate alcohol consumption and risk of heart failure among older persons. JAMA 2001;285:1971–7.
35. Walsh CR, Larson MG, Evans JC, et al. Alcohol consumption and risk for congestive heart failure in the Framingham Heart Study. Ann Intern Med 2002;136: 181–91.
36. Piepoli MF, Davos C, Francis DP, et al. Exercise training meta-analysis of trials in patients with chronic heart failure (ExTraMATCH). BMJ 2004;328:189.

37. Wilson JR, Reichek N, Dunkman WB, et al. Effect of diuresis on the performance of the failing left ventricle in man. Am J Med 1981;70:234–9.

38. Parker JO. The effects of oral ibopamine in patients with mild heart failure: a double blind placebo controlled comparison to furosemide: the Ibopamine Study Group. Int J Cardiol 1993;40:221–7.

39. Richardson A, Bayliss J, Scriven AJ, et al. Double-blind comparison of captopril alone against frusemide plus amiloride in mild heart failure. Lancet 1987;2: 709–11.

40. Pitt B, Zannad F, Remme WJ, et al. The effect of spironolactone on morbidity and mortality in patients with severe heart failure. Randomized Aldactone Evaluation Study Investigators. N Engl J Med 1999;341:709–17.

41. Zannad F, McMurray JJ, Krum H, et al. Eplerenone in patients with systolic heart failure and mild symptoms. N Engl J Med 2011;364:11–21.

42. Makani H, Messerli FH, Romero J, et al. Meta-analysis of randomized trials of angioedema as an adverse event of renin-angiotensin system inhibitors. Am J Cardiol 2012;110:383–91.

43. Toh S, Reichman ME, Houstoun M, et al. Comparative risk for angioedema associated with the use of drugs that target the renin-angiotensin-aldosterone system. Arch Intern Med 2012;172:1582–9.

44. Pfeffer MA, McMurray JJ, Velazquez EJ, et al. Valsartan, captopril, or both in myocardial infarction complicated by heart failure, left ventricular dysfunction, or both. N Engl J Med 2003;349:1893–906.

45. Granger CB, McMurray JJ, Yusuf S, et al. Effects of candesartan in patients with chronic heart failure and reduced left-ventricular systolic function intolerant to angiotensin-converting-enzyme inhibitors: the CHARM-Alternative trial. Lancet 2003;362:772–6.

46. Packer M, Coats AJ, Fowler MB, et al. Effect of carvedilol on survival in severe chronic heart failure. N Engl J Med 2001;344:1651–8.

47. Effect of metoprolol CR/XL in chronic heart failure: metoprolol CR/XL randomised intervention trial in congestive heart failure (MERIT-HF). Lancet 1999;353:2001–7.

48. Guyatt GH, Sullivan MJ, Fallen EL, et al. A controlled trial of digoxin in congestive heart failure. Am J Cardiol 1988;61:371–5.

49. Uretsky BF, Young JB, Shahidi FE, et al. Randomized study assessing the effect of digoxin withdrawal in patients with mild to moderate chronic congestive heart failure: results of the PROVED trial: PROVED Investigative Group. J Am Coll Cardiol 1993;22:955–62.

50. Taylor AL, Ziesche S, Yancy C, et al. Combination of isosorbide dinitrate and hydralazine in blacks with heart failure. N Engl J Med 2004;351:2049–57.

51. Felker GM, O'Connor CM. Inotropic therapy for heart failure: an evidence-based approach. Am Heart J 2001;142:393–401.

52. Cuffe MS, Califf RM, Adams KF, et al, for the Outcomes of a Prospective Trial of Intravenous Milrinone for Exacerbations of Chronic Heart Failure (OPTIME-CHF) Investigators. Short-term intravenous milrinone for acute exacerbation of chronic heart failure: a randomized controlled trial. JAMA 2002; 287:1541–7.

53. Dickstein K, Cohen-Solal A, Filippatos G, et al. ESC guidelines for the diagnosis and treatment of acute and chronic heart failure 2008: the Task Force for the Diagnosis and Treatment of Acute and Chronic Heart Failure 2008 of the European Society of Cardiology: developed in collaboration with the Heart Failure Association of the ESC (HFA) and endorsed by the European Society of Intensive Care Medicine (ESICM). Eur Heart J 2008;29:2388–442.

54. Maisel WH, Stevenson LW. Atrial fibrillation in heart failure: epidemiology, patho-physiology, and rationale for therapy. Am J Cardiol 2003;91:2D–8D.
55. McMurray JJ, Packer M, Desai AS, et al. Dual angiotensin receptor and neprilysin inhibition as an alternative to angiotensin-converting enzyme inhibition in patients with chronic systolic heart failure: rationale for and design of the Prospective comparison of ARNI with ACEI to Determine Impact on Global Mortality and morbidity in Heart Failure trial (PARADIGM-HF). Eur J Heart Fail 2013;15(9):1062–73.
56. Böhm M, Borer J, Ford I, et al. Heart rate at baseline influences the effect of ivab-radine on cardiovascular outcomes in chronic heart failure: analysis from the SHIFT study. Clin Res Cardiol 2013;102(1):11–22.
57. O'Connor CM, Starling RC, Hernandez AF, et al. Effect of nesiritide in patients with acute decompensated heart failure. N Engl J Med 2011;365:32–43.
58. Hernandez A, O'Connor CM, Starling RC, et al. Rationale and design of the Acute Study of Clinical Effectiveness of Nesiritide in Decompensated Heart Failure trial (ASCEND-HF). Am Heart J 2009;157(2):271–7.
59. Nohria A, Desai A. Reducing readmissions with novel cardiac resynchronization therapy programming. J Am Coll Cardiol 2015;3(7):573–5.
60. Moss AJ, Hall WJ, Cannom DS, et al. Cardiac-resynchronization therapy for the prevention of heart-failure events. N Engl J Med 2009;361:1329–38.
61. Tang AS, Wells GA, Talajic M, et al. Cardiac-resynchronization therapy for mild-to-moderate heart failure. N Engl J Med 2010;363:2385–95.
62. Elhenawy AM, Algarni KD, Rodger M, et al. Mechanical circulatory support as a bridge to transplant candidacy. J Cardiovasc Surg 2011;26:542–7.
63. Nair PK, Kormos RL, Teuteberg JJ, et al. Pulsatile left ventricular assist device support as a bridge to decision in patients with end-stage heart failure compli-cated by pulmonary hypertension. J Heart Lung Transplant 2010;29:201–8.
64. Miller LW, Pagani FD, Russell SD, et al. Use of a continuous-flow device in patients awaiting heart transplantation. N Engl J Med 2007;357:885–96.
65. Stehlik J, Edwards LB, Kucheryavaya AY, et al. The Registry of the International Society for Heart and Lung Transplantation: twenty-eighth adult heart transplant report–2011. J Heart Lung Transplant 2011;30:1078–94.
66. Goda A, Lund LH, Mancini D. The heart failure survival score outperforms the peak oxygen consumption for heart transplantation selection in the era of device therapy. J Heart Lung Transplant 2011;30:315–25.
67. Hunt SA. ACC/AHA 2005 guidelines for the diagnosis and management of chronic heart failure in the adult: a report of the American College of Cardiol-ogy/American Heart Association Task Force on Practice Guidelines (Writing Com-mittee to Update the 2001 Guidelines for the Evaluation and Management of Heart Failure). J Am Coll Cardiol 2005;46:e1–82. Current ACC/AHA practice guidelines including comprehensive overview of the literature until 2005, together with references 1 and 2.
68. Friedrich E, Bohm M. Management of end stage heart failure. Heart 2007;93(5):626–31.

Platelet Inhibitors

Megan M. Shifrin, DNP, RN, ACNP-BC[a],*,
S. Brian Widmar, PhD, RN, ACNP-BC, CCRN[b],*

KEYWORDS

- Nursing • Acute coronary syndrome • Platelets • Antiplatelet • Thrombosis
- Bleeding

KEY POINTS

- Antithrombotic medications have become standard of care for management of acute coronary syndromes (ACSs).
- Platelet adhesion, activation, and aggregation are essential components of platelet function; platelet-inhibiting medications interfere with these components and reduce incidence of thrombosis.
- Active bleeding is a contraindication for administration of platelet inhibitors.
- There is currently no reversal agent for platelet inhibitors, although platelet transfusion may be used to correct active bleeding after administration of platelet inhibitors.

INTRODUCTION

Platelets are an essential part of a complex protective pathway used by the body to maintain hemostasis. After adhering to the site of vascular injury, platelets activate and secrete substances that attract other platelets, resulting in an aggregation of platelets around the site of injury in an attempt to stop acute blood loss. Under some pathologic conditions, such as atherosclerosis and inflammatory disorders, this process leads to thrombosis and arterial occlusion. Subsequently, a variety of potential complications may result, including life-threatening conditions, such as ACSs.[1] According to recent statistics provided by the American Heart Association, an estimated 15.5 million Americans 20 years of age or older has coronary heart disease.[2] The American Heart Association also projects that, based on available research, 635,000 Americans will have a new coronary event, and another 300,000 will have a recurrent event.[2]

Strategies used to reduce risk of thrombosis in ACSs include antiplatelet agents, such as antithrombin drugs (eg, unfractionated and low-molecular-weight heparin

Disclosures: None.
[a] Vanderbilt University School of Nursing, 461 21st Avenue South, 382 Frist Hall, Nashville, TN 37240, USA; [b] Vanderbilt University School of Nursing, 461 21st Avenue South, 366 Frist Hall, Nashville, TN 37240, USA
* Corresponding authors.
E-mail addresses: megan.m.tyser@vanderbilt.edu; brian.widmar@vanderbilt.edu

and direct thrombin inhibitors), aspirin, thienopyridines, and glycoprotein (Gp)IIb/IIIa inhibitors.[3] Previous trials evaluating the use of oral antiplatelet agents in ACSs have supported the combined administration of thienopyridines and aspirin; current standards include a course of treatment of up to 1 year after an ACS event.[3] This article discusses platelet formation and life cycle, the antiplatelet medications most commonly used in the treatment of ACSs, and guidelines for drug administration and implications for nursing care.

PLATELET FORMATION AND LIFE CYCLE

Functional platelets are developed through the intricate process of thrombopoesis. Thrombopoietin, a Gp hormone produced by sinusoidal and parenchymal cells in the liver and proximal convoluted tubule cells kidneys, is responsible for regulating the growth, number, and differentiation of megakaryocytes in the bone marrow.[4–6] These progenitor cells extend small budlike pseudopodia into the bone marrow sinusoids, releasing anucleate cell fragments that migrate into systemic circulation.[7] Platelets undergo their final maturation processes while circulating in the blood stream, although there are some data to support that the pulmonary system may be involved in this process as well.[8] Once fully mature, the average lifetime of a disk-shaped platelet is approximately 8 to 10 days.[9]

PLATELET FUNCTION

Platelets are commonly associated with their involvement in thrombosis and hemostasis; however, they also plan significant roles in inflammation and immunity.[10] The primary insult triggering a platelet response is vascular injury involving the intimal layer of the blood vessel. After vascular compromise, the stepwise process of platelet adhesion, activation, and aggregation occurs to protect the host from further physiologic consequences. For the purpose of this article, the discussion of pathways involved in these processes is largely limited to those directly associated with pharmacologic platelet inhibitor management.

ADHESION

Vascular injury can stem from multiple sources; atherosclerosis, sheer force, and direct vessel compromise, however, remain the primary mechanisms through which platelets are activated. Damaged vascular endothelium exposes platelets to both activated von Willebrand factor (vWF) and collagen in subendothelium, triggering 2 simultaneous mechanisms that are foundational for platelet adhesion to the site of injury (**Fig. 1**). The first process takes place when activated vWF binds with GpIb-V-IX complex, a receptor on the platelet cell membrane. The second process occurs when exposed collagen from damaged endothelial cells binds with platelet GpVI, a separate receptor on the platelet cell membrane. Collaboratively, these processes work to tether the platelet to the site of vascular injury.[1,11]

ACTIVATION

Once the platelet has been bound to the site of injury, activation of the platelet occurs (**Fig. 2**). The activated platelet releases several mediators, including ADP, thromboxane A_2 (TxA_2), and thrombin. ADP amplifies platelet activation and recruits additional platelets to the site of compromise to achieve hemostasis.[12] Additionally, ADP is instrumental in changing the morphology of the platelet from its disklike shape

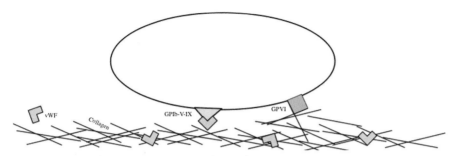

Fig. 1. Adhesion of platelets to the site of vascular injury.

to an amorphous shape with multiple finger-like projections to increase platelet surface area and optimize the coagulation process.[1,13]

TxA$_2$ enhances thrombus formation through 2 different mechanisms. First, TxA$_2$ serves as a potent vasoconstrictor when released from the platelet.[14] Second, TxA$_2$ causes an increase in the expression of GpIIb/IIIa complexes on the surface of platelet.[13]

Cyclic adenosine monophosphate (cAMP) and cyclic guanosine monophosphate (cGMP) are secondary messengers responsible for signaling within the platelet. cAMP and cGMP are responsible for regulating key aspects of platelet activation and aggregation. Intraplatelet cAMP and cGMP are degraded by an enzyme called phosphodiesterase (PDE).[15]

AGGREGATION

The process of platelet accumulation at the site of the vascular injury begins after expression and activation of GpIIb/IIIa complexes (**Fig. 3**). Fibrinogen and vWF essentially serve as connecting links that join circulating platelets together. As the cumulative binding of platelet GpIIa/IIIb with circulating fibrinogen strands and

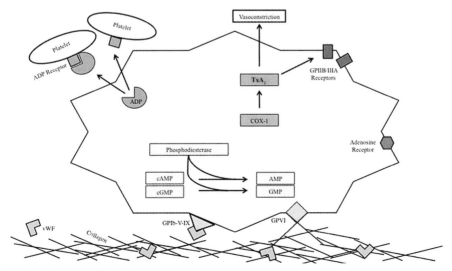

Fig. 2. Activation of platelets.

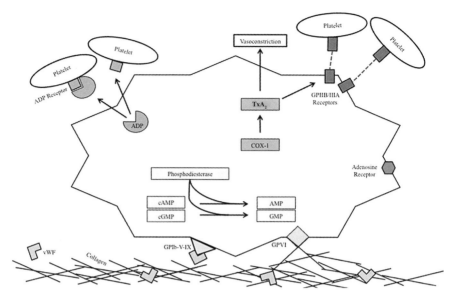

Fig. 3. Aggregation of platelets at the site of injury.

vWF in the plasma occur, the platelet plug continues to grow and contribute to hemostasis.[11]

PHARMACOLOGIC PLATELET INHIBITORS

Pharmacologic platelet inhibitors consist of several different agents that each act differently in the platelet adhesion-activation-aggregation progression (**Fig. 4**).

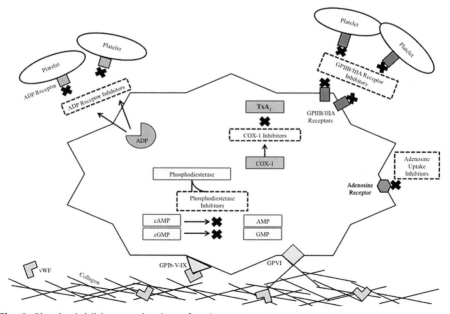

Fig. 4. Platelet inhibitor mechanism of action.

Interruption of platelet intracellular signaling pathways and blockade of ligand receptors on the platelet membrane are the primary mechanisms of action of medications in
this class. Individually or collaboratively, these medications function to alter platelet
activation and aggregation, thus making affected platelets less thrombotic in nature.
Specific indications for pharmacologic therapy and dosing recommendations are
found in **Table 1**.

CYCLOOXYGENASE-1 INHIBITORS: ASPIRIN

Aspirin is the most used platelet inhibitor globally due to its efficacy, availability, and
affordability. The Food and Drug Administration (FDA) has approved aspirin for use
in patients as secondary prevention in several different cardiovascular disease states.
Additionally, aspirin may be used after procedures associated with revascularization
(see **Table 1**). Some data have suggested that aspirin may be beneficial in the primary
prevention of myocardial infarction and stroke. The FDA, however, has not approved
aspirin for use in this capacity.[16] Aspirin comes in both oral and rectal suppository
preparations, although oral dosing is the preferred method of administration. Aspirin
doses range from 81 mg to 650 mg daily depending on a patient's medical indications
and comorbid conditions (see **Table 1**).

Mechanism of Action

Aspirin irreversibly acetylates cyclooxygenase-1 (COX-1) and inhibits the formation of
prostaglandin H2. As a result, platelets are unable to produce TxA_2 and generate additional GpIIb/IIIa complexes on the surface of platelet. Subsequently, vasodilation and
platelet aggregation are prohibited.

Pharmacokinetics

Aspirin is primarily absorbed through the gastrointestinal tract. Rates of aspirin absorption vary based on the gastrointestinal pH, presence of buffering agents, and
the medication dose and preparation. Aspirin is primarily hydrolyzed in the plasma
to form salicylic acid and then further metabolized in the liver to form salicyluric
acid.[17] Urinary pH directly affects the renal excretion of aspirin. Excretion rates are
higher in environments where the urinary pH is greater than 6.5.[18]

Contraindications

Aspirin should not be administered to people with a history of hypersensitivity or allergy to nonsteroidal anti-inflammatory drugs (NSAIDs) because this may result in hypersensitivity reactions, such as urticaria, asthma, and angioedema.[18] It should not be
administered to patients with suspected viral illnesses due to the risk of Reye syndrome.[17] In patients with anemia, hemophilia, thrombocytopenia, ongoing bleeding
disorders, and gastrointestinal disorders, such as peptic ulcer disease and ulcerative
colitis, the use of aspirin may lead increased bleeding and bleeding times due to
platelet function inhibition.[17]

PHOSPHODIESTERASE INHIBITORS: CILOSTAZOL

Cilostazol has been FDA approved for use in patients with peripheral arterial disease
and intermittent claudication.[18] Cilostazol has also been studied in multiple other
vascular disease states and continues to be used in an off-label manner.

A reduced dose of cilostazol should be considered when patients are taking other
medications that are metabolized via the same hepatic pathways.[19] Some of these

Table 1
Platelet-inhibiting medications

Drug Name	Indication for Use	Dosing Recommendations	Reversal/Half-Life	Nursing Implications
COX-1 inhibitors[16,17]				
Aspirin	• Ischemic stroke • Transient ischemic attack • Suspected acute MI • Stable chronic angina pectoris • UA pectoris • Prevention of recurrent MI • CAB grafting • Percutaneous transluminal coronary angioplasty • Carotid endarterectomy	• 50–325 mg orally once daily • Continue therapy indefinitely 160–162.5 mg orally once on symptom onset • 75–325 mg orally once daily • Continue therapy indefinitely • 325 mg orally once daily starting 6 h postprocedure • Continue therapy for 1 y postprocedure • Initial dose of 325 mg orally given 2 h prior to the procedure • Maintenance dose of 160–325 mg orally once daily • Continue therapy indefinitely • 80 mg orally once daily to 650 mg orally every 12 h starting prior to surgery • Continue therapy indefinitely	• No reversal agent • Effects last for the life of the platelet • With profound bleeding, platelet transfusion may be indicated • Desmopressin 0.3 mg/kg IV × 1 may provide some coagulation benefit	• Provide with food to decrease GI upset • Adjust dose in severe hepatic failure • Education includes monitoring for signs/symptoms of anemia and GI bleeding, tinnitus or hearing loss

PDE inhibitors[18,19,22,23]

Drug	Indications	Dosing	Reversal	Side effects / Education
Cilostazol	• Peripheral arterial disease • Intermittent claudication	100 mg orally every 12 h taken 30 min prior to a meal or 2 h after a meal	No reversal agent	• Most common side effect is headache • Serious side effects include heart failure, GI bleed, and atrial fibrillation • Education includes monitoring for peripheral edema, dyspnea, melena, and anemia

Adenosine reuptake inhibitors[26-28]

Drug	Indications	Dosing	Reversal	Side effects / Education
Dipyridamole	• Prosthetic heart valve • Implanted cardiac ventricular assist device	75–100 mg orally every 6 h	• No reversal agent • Effects last for the life of the platelet • With profound bleeding, platelet transfusion may be indicated • Desmopressin 0.3 mg/kg IV × 1 may provide some coagulation benefit	• Headache is common and may require dose adjustment • Increased risk for ICH and GI bleeding • Use cautiously in patients with renal failure • Avoid in pregnancy • Signs of overdose include flushing, diaphoresis, weakness, dizziness, and hypotension
Aspirin/dipyridamole extended-release	Transient ischemic attack or ischemic stroke due to thrombosis	Aspirin 25 mg/dipyridamole extended-release 200 mg orally every 12 h		

(continued on next page)

Table 1
(continued)

Drug Name	Indication for Use	Dosing Recommendations	Reversal/Half-Life	Nursing Implications
GpIIb/IIIa receptor antagonists[29,30]				
Abciximab	Prevention of cardiac ischemia in patients with ACSs treated with PCI, and in patients with UA refractory to standard therapy up to 24 h prior to PCI	• PCI: 0.25-mg/kg IV bolus 10–60 min before PCI, followed by infusion of 0.125 μg/kg/min for 12 h • UA refractory to medical therapy, within 24 h of PCI: 0.25-mg/kg IV bolus, followed by 18–24 h infusion of 10 μg/min. Stop infusion 1 h after PCI	• With profound bleeding, action can be reversed by platelet transfusion • Half-life 30 min	• Most common complications include bleeding (GI, genitourinary, arterial catheterization sites, peripheral venipuncture sites, etc.) • Minimize venipuncture and injections once infusions have been initiated • Use in extreme caution when platelet count is <150,000/mm^3
Eptifibatide	Prevention of cardiac ischemia in patients with ACSs treated with either medical management or PCI	• ACSs: 180-μg/kg IV bolus (maximum 22.6 mg) over 1–2 min Follow with 2-μg/kg/min infusion (maximum 15 mg/h) up to 72 h, or until CAB • PCI with or without stent: 180-μg/kg IV bolus (maximum 22.6 mg) immediately before PCI Repeat bolus 10 min after first bolus is given. Follow with 2-μg/kg/min infusion (maximum 15 mg/h) up to 18–24 h	• Considered reversible as platelet function returns to normal within 6 h after discontinuation of infusion • Half-life 2.5 h	
Tirofiban	Prevention of cardiac ischemia in patients with ACSs treated with either medical management or PCI	ACSs: begin IV infusion at 0.4 μg/kg/min for 30 min, then continue at 0.1 μg/kg/min Continue during and for 12–24 h after PCI	• Considered reversible as platelet function returns to normal within 6 h after discontinuation of infusion • Half-life 2 h	

ADP receptor inhibitors[3,29–31]

Drug	Uses	Dosing	Reversal	Comments
Clopidogrel	• Reduction of atherosclerotic events in patients with recent ACSs, stroke, or PAD • ACS with PCI (with/without stent) or CAB • STEMI treated by fibrinolysis and aspirin • Prevention of late poststent thrombosis after BMSs or DESs • Aspirin resistance	• PCI in low- to moderate-risk patients; urgent PCI in high-risk ACSs patients without STEMI: 600-mg oral loading dose • UA/NSTEMI: 300-mg oral loading dose, followed by 75 mg daily • STEMI: 75 mg orally daily (taken in addition to aspirin) • Prevention of late poststent thrombosis after BMS/DES: 75 mg orally daily for at least 12 mo • Aspirin resistance: 75 mg orally daily may be used to substitute for aspirin	• No reversal agent • Effects last for the life of the platelet • With profound bleeding, platelet transfusion may be indicated	• Proton pump inhibitors inhibit conversion of clopidogrel to its active form and reduces efficacy • Discontinue therapy 5 d prior to CAB if possible • Monitor for increased bleeding Active bleeding is a contraindication for use
Prasugrel	Reduction of atherosclerotic events in patients with recent ACSs (UA, NSTEMI, or STEMI) treated with PCI (with/without stent)	• Loading dose: 60 mg orally daily, no later than 1 h after PCI • Maintenance: 10 mg orally daily for 12–15 mo • Duration: 10 mg orally daily for 12 mo after BMS/DES	• No reversal agent • With profound bleeding, platelet transfusion may be indicated	• Often used when patient is resistant to clopidogrel • Not used with fibrinolytic therapy or in patients without PCI • Elimination half-life of approximately 7 h Platelet aggregation returns to baseline within 5–9 d • Monitor for increased bleeding Active bleeding is a contraindication for use

(continued on next page)

Table 1
(continued)

Drug Name	Indication for Use	Dosing Recommendations	Reversal/Half-Life	Nursing Implications
Ticagrelor	Secondary prevention of thrombotic events after ACSs managed with or without PCI or CAB	• Loading dose: 180 mg orally • Maintenance: 90 mg orally twice daily starting 12 h after loading dose	• No reversal agent • Half-life of 7 h for parent drug and 9 h for active metabolite	• Increased risk of bleeding • Most common side effects are dyspnea and bleeding
Cangrelor	Secondary prevention of thrombotic events after ACSs in patients undergoing PCI	• Loading dose: 30-μg/kg IV bolus infused over 1 min before PCI • Maintenance: 4-μg/kg/min IV infusion, continue for at least 2 h or duration of PCI, whichever is longer	Immediate effects and short half-life (2–3 min)	Increased risk of bleeding, greater than with clopidogrel

Abbreviations: BMS, bare metal stent; CAB, coronary artery bypass; DES, drug-eluting stent; GI, gastrointestinal; ICH, intracranial hemorrhage; IV, intravenous; MI, myocardial infarction; NSTEMI, non–ST segment elevation myocardial infarction, STEMI, ST segment elevation myocardial infarction; UA, unstable angina.

medications include ketoconazole, itraconazole, fluconazole, erythromycin, diltiazem, and omeprazole.

Mechanism of Action

Collectively, PDE-inhibiting medications block PDE from participating within metabolic pathways in the platelet. As a result, intraplatelet cAMP concentrations rise, which subsequently impede platelet aggregation properties.[20] Cilostazol is responsible for inhibiting PDE3, a specific PDE. PDE inhibition also results in vasodilation of peripheral tissues.[21]

Pharmacokinetics

Cilostazol is absorbed from the gastrointestinal system. Because high-fat meals increase the cilostazol concentration-time curve, cilostazol should be taken on an empty stomach 30 minutes prior to a meal or 2 hours after meals.[21] Cilostazol is primarily protein-bound to albumin in the plasma; thus, nutritional state may play a role in cilostazol serum concentrations. Cilostazol is metabolized through the hepatic system.[20] Elimination of the cilostazol occurs primarily via the renal system; however, up to 20% of cilostazol metabolites have been found in feces. No adjustments to dosing need to be made for patients with renal insufficiency.[20]

Contraindications

The FDA has issued a black box warning for the use of cilostazol in all heart failure patients because similar PDE inhibitors have increased mortality in heart failure populations.[22] Cilostazol is also contraindicated for use in patients who have ongoing pathologic bleeding, such as patients with a gastric ulcer or intracranial hemorrhage.[21]

ADENOSINE REUPTAKE INHIBITORS: DIPYRIDAMOLE

When used in conjunction with warfarin, it has been shown to decrease thromboembolic events in patients with artificial heart valves.[23] It is also used as a form of anticoagulation in patients who have received implanted ventricular assist devices.[24]

Extended-release dipyridamole also comes prepared in combination with aspirin and is FDA approved as a form of secondary prevention in patients who have a history of transient ischemic attack or ischemic stroke associated with thrombosis.[25]

Mechanism of Action

Dipyridamole exhibits multiple mechanisms of action. The primary effect of dipyridamole comes from the inhibition of adenosine reuptake in platelets and erythrocytes, thus increasing the extracellular plasma concentration of adenosine and causing systemic vasodilation. This effect is dependent on the dipyridamole concentration in whole blood.[26] Second, dipyridamole is a weak PDE inhibitor (PDE3 and PDE5). In response to PDE inhibition, intraplatelet cAMP and cGMP concentrations increase. Heightened presence of these intracellular messengers prevent the platelet from exhibiting many of the functions necessary for platelet adhesion and aggregation.[27] Lastly, dipyridamole serves as an antioxidant that may reduce thrombotic activity through the reducing damage caused by reactive oxidative species.[28]

Pharmacokinetics

Dipyridamole is absorbed in the gastrointestinal system and then metabolized in the liver. Peak plasma levels typically occur 2 hours after administration. A majority of dipyridamole metabolites are excreted into bile and then ultimately eliminated into the feces. Renal and urinary excretion of dipyridamole metabolites is low (approximately 5%). Because dipyridamole is prepared in combination with aspirin, however, renal and urinary clearance should also be considered.

Contraindications

Aspirin/dipyridamole should not be administered to people with a history of asthma in combination with rhinitis and nasal polyps, hypersensitivity, or allergies to NSAIDs because this may result in hypersensitivity reactions, such as urticaria, asthma exacerbations, and angioedema.[25] Due to the aspirin component in the medication combination, it should not be administered to patients with suspected viral illnesses due to the risk of Reye syndrome.[25] In patients with anemia, hemophilia, thrombocytopenia, ongoing bleeding disorders, and gastrointestinal disorders, such as peptic ulcer disease and ulcerative colitis, the use of aspirin/dipyridamole may lead increased bleeding and bleeding times due to platelet function inhibition.

GLYCOPROTEIN IIb/IIIa RECEPTOR ANTAGONISTS: ABCIXIMAB, EPTIFIBATIDE, AND TIROFIBAN

The 3 most commonly cited GpIIb/IIIa inhibitors are abciximab, tirofiban, and eptifibatide. All have been studied when used in conjunction with aspirin and/or antithrombotic therapy, but studies occurred prior to the routine use of thienopyridines.[29]

Mechanism of Action

GpIIb/IIIa receptor antagonists inhibit platelet aggregation by binding to the GpIIb/IIIa receptors on platelets, preventing fibrinogen from binding to platelets and rendering them unable to cross-link.[29,30] Through this mechanism, GpIIb/IIIa receptor antagonists may give added protection to patients with ACSs who are also treated with other antiplatelet agents and thrombolytics.[29]

Pharmacokinetics

Abciximab is a monoclonal antibody against the platelet GpIIb/IIIa receptor. Its inhibition of platelet aggregation peaks 2 hours after a bolus is administered and returns to normal after 12 hours.[29] The antibody can be transmitted to new platelets and can be detected up to 14 days after administration.[29]

Tirofiban is a nonpeptide petidomimetic GpIIb/IIIa inhibitor and is less likely to cause a hypersensitivity reaction than abciximab.[29] It has an acute onset and its half-life is approximately 2 hours. Eptifibatide is a synthetic cyclic heptapeptide that binds at a different site on the GpIIb/IIIa receptor than tirofiban, and it also has a lesser likelihood of hypersensitivity reaction than abciximab.[29] Eptifibatide's affinity for its receptor is lower than those of abciximab and tirofiban; epitifibatide requires a higher dose for optimal efficacy.[29] The half-life of eptifibatide is approximately 2 hours.[30]

Contraindications

Most contraindications to GpIIb/IIIa inhibitors involve acute bleeding, high risk for acute bleeding, or preexisting thrombocytopenia. One of the most commonly reported complications of GpIIb/IIIa inhibitors is increased bleeding at the cardiac catheterization arterial access site.[29] All GpIIb/IIIa inhibitors require dose adjustments in the setting of renal disease, and abciximab has an increased likelihood of hypersensitivity reaction.[29,30]

ADENOSINE DIPHOSPHATE INHIBITORS: CLOPIDOGREL, PRASUGREL, TICAGRELOR, AND CANGRELOR
Mechanism of Action

Clopidogrel, prasugrel, ticagrelor, and cangrelor are thienopyridines that are ADP inhibitors; they act at a different site from aspirin, irreversibly inhibiting the binding of platelet ADP to the $P2Y_{12}$ receptor.[29] Through this process, transformation and activation of the GpIIb/IIIa receptor are prevented.[29,30]

Pharmacokinetics

Clopidogrel is a prodrug with a slow onset of action. It requires conversion to its active form by the liver.[30] The onset of action on platelets is within hours of the first dose, with steady state inhibition occurring at approximately 3 to 7 days. Maximal inhibition is achieved by loading dose (see **Table 1**). Inhibition lasts for the life of the platelet.[30]

  Prasugrel is also a prodrug, and it is metabolized into both active and inactive metabolites. It has enhanced hepatic conversion, so its active metabolites have a more rapid onset and greater effect on both platelet activation and aggregation than clopidogrel.[29] Platelet aggregation returns to baseline after 5 to 9 days of discontinuation.[30] Ticagrelor reversibly binds to ADP receptors and prevents platelet activation and reduces aggregation. The parent drug has a half-life of approximately 7 hours, whereas the active metabolite has a half-life of 9 hours.[30] Cangrelor recently received approval by the FDA for use in adult patients undergoing percutaneous coronary intervention (PCI). Delivered intravenously before and during the PCI procedure, it rapidly achieves steady state concentrations and has a half-life of 2 to 3 minutes. After cessation of the infusion, it is rapidly removed, resulting in restoration of normal platelet function in approximately an hour.[31]

Contraindications

Thienopyridines are contraindicated in patients with active bleeding (eg, peptic ulcer disease or intracranial hemorrhage) or in patients with coagulation disorders.[29]

SUMMARY

Platelet inhibitors play a critical role in the pharmacologic management of cardiovascular disease processes and are effective in decreasing morbidity and mortality associated with many cardiovascular disease states by ideally preventing thrombosis while also achieving hemostasis. Platelet inhibitors also remain valued in cardiovascular treatment profiles due to their ease of administration, affordability, and rapid onset of action. The lack of reversal agents, however, remains a drawback to use.

  Prior to administering an antiplatelet medication, health care providers should evaluate a patient's past medical history and allergies to decrease the potential of adverse drug events. Bleeding continues to remain one of the most problematic complications that results from antiplatelet drug administration; however, patient education regarding prescribed medication administration, dosing, therapeutic evaluation, and adverse events can play a pivotal role in reducing morbidity and mortality associated with this problem. Due to the rapid onset of action associated with intravenous inhibitors, nurses should be vigilant in evaluating for signs and symptoms of bleeding diathesis when performing patient physical assessments and monitoring. Future research should be directed at identifying reversal agents for rapid offset of action, further evaluating the role of genetics and medication efficacy, and refining strategies for medication safety.

REFERENCES

1. Furie B, Furie BC. Mechanisms of thrombus formation. N Engl J Med 2008;359(9): 938–49.
2. Mozaffarian D, Benjamin EJ, Go AS, et al. Heart disease and stroke statistics–2015 update: a report from the American Heart Association. Circulation 2015; 131(4):e29–322.
3. Birkeland K, Parra D, Rosenstein R. Antiplatelet therapy in acute coronary syndromes: focus on ticagrelor. J Blood Med 2010;1:197–219.
4. Kaushansky K. Thrombopoetin: the primary regulator of platelet production. Blood 1995;85:419–31.
5. Kopp HG, Avecilla ST, Hooper AT, et al. The bone marrow vascular niche: home of HSC differentiation and mobilization. Physiology (Bethesda) 2005;20:349–56.
6. Machlus KR, Italiano JE Jr. The incredible journey: From megakaryocyte development to platelet formation. J Cell Biol 2013;201(6):785–96.
7. Tavassoli M, Aoki M. Localization of megakaryocytes in the bone marrow. Blood Cells 1989;15(1):3–14.
8. Trowbridge EA, Martin JF, Slater DN. Evidence for a theory of physical fragmentation of megakaryocytes, implying that all platelets are produced in the pulmonary circulation. Thromb Res 1982;28(4):461–75.
9. Harker LA, Roskos LK, Marzec UM, et al. Effects of megakaryocyte growth and development factor on platelet production, platelet life span, and platelet function in healthy human volunteers. Blood 2000;95(8):2514–22.
10. Ross R. Atherosclerosis–an inflammatory disease. N Engl J Med 1999;340(2): 115–26.
11. Ruggeri ZM. Platelets in atherothrombosis. Nat Med 2002;8(11):1227–34.
12. Davi G, Patrono C. Platelet activation and atherothrombosis. N Engl J Med 2007; 357(24):2482–94.
13. Wilde JI, Retzer M, Siess W, et al. ADP-induced platelet shape change: an investigation of the signalling pathways involved and their dependence on the method of platelet preparation. Platelets 2000;11(5):286–95.
14. Reilly M, Fitzgerald GA. Cellular activation by thromboxane A2 and other eicosanoids. Eur Heart J 1993;14(Suppl K):88–93.
15. Smolenski A. Novel roles of cAMP/cGMP-dependent signaling in platelets. J Thromb Haemost 2012;10(2):167–76.
16. Use of aspirin for primary prevention of heart attack and stroke. Available at: http://www.fda.gov/Drugs/ResourcesForYou/Consumers/ucm390574.htm. Accessed June 12, 2015.
17. Aspirin: Comprehensive prescribing information. Available at: http://www.fda.gov/ohrms/DOCKETS/ac/03/briefing/4012B1_03_Appd 1-Professional Labeling.pdf. Accessed June 14, 2015.
18. Kumar M, Bhattacharya V. Cilostazol: a new drug in the treatment intermittent claudication. Recent Pat Cardiovasc Drug Discov 2007;2(3):181–5.
19. Bramer S, Tata P, Mallikaarjun S. Disposition of 14 C-cilostazol after single dose administration to healthy human subjects. Pharmacol Res 1997;14(11 Suppl):S612.
20. Ji X, Hou M. Novel agents for anti-platelet therapy. J Hematol Oncol 2011;4:44.
21. Rogers KC, Oliphant CS, Finks SW. Clinical efficacy and safety of cilostazol: a critical review of the literature. Drugs 2015;75(4):377–95.
22. Packer M, Carver JR, Rodeheffer RJ, et al. Effect of oral milrinone on mortality in severe chronic heart failure. The PROMISE Study Research Group. N Engl J Med 1991;325(21):1468–75.

23. Massel DR, Little SH. Antiplatelet and anticoagulation for patients with prosthetic heart valves. Cochrane Database Syst Rev 2013;(7):CD003464.
24. Russell S, Slaughter M, Pagani F, et al. HMII LVAS guidelines. Available at: http://www.fda.gov/ohrms/DOCKETS/ac/07/briefing/2007-4333b2-20-9_4 HM II Patient Management Guidelines.pdf. Accessed June 11, 2015.
25. Aggrenox prescribing information. Available at: http://www.accessdata.fda.gov/drugsatfda_docs/label/2012/020884s030lbl.pdf. Accessed June 15, 2015.
26. Klabunde RE. Dipyridamole inhibition of adenosine metabolism in human blood. Eur J Pharmacol 1993;93:21–6.
27. Harker LA, Kadatz RA. Mechanism of action of dipyridamole. Thromb Res Suppl 1983;4:39–46.
28. Parthasarathy S, Steinberg D, Witztum JL. The role of oxidized low-density lipoproteins in the pathogenesis of atherosclerosis. Annu Rev Med 1992;43:219–25.
29. Fox KA, White H, Opie JJ, et al. Antithrombotic agents: platelet inhibitors, anticoagulants, and fibrinolytics. In: Opie LH, Gersh BJ, editors. Drugs for the heart. 7th edition. Philadelphia: Saunders; 2009. p. 293–340.
30. Jacobson C, Marzlin K, Webner C. 2nd edition. Cardiovascular nursing practice: a comprehensive resource manual and study guide for clinical nurses, vol. 2. Burien (WA): Cardiovascular Education Associates; 2014.
31. Kubica J, Kozinski M, Navarese EP, et al. Cangrelor: an emerging therapeutic option for patients with coronary artery disease. Curr Med Res Opin 2014;30(5):813–28.

Updates on the Pharmacologic Treatment of Individuals with Human Immunodeficiency Virus

Courtney J. Young, DNP, MPH, FNP-BC

KEYWORDS

- Human immunodeficiency virus • Antiretroviral therapy • Adults • Children
- Pregnancy

KEY POINTS

- HIV has been affecting the human population for more than 30 years.
- To date, there are 26 antiretroviral agents available which are used either as a single agent or a co-formulation in an antiretroviral regimen.
- The goal of these medications is to achieve viral suppression in individuals infected with HIV.
- It is of utter importance that clinicians are knowledgeable of updates so as to provide the best possible medical regimen for those affected by HIV.

INTRODUCTION

According to the Centers for Disease Control and Prevention, an estimated 47,500 individuals became infected with human immunodeficiency virus (HIV) in 2010.[1] Although the incidence of new HIV cases has plateaued around 50,000 since the mid-1990s, it is notable that there has been a decreasing trend in new cases among African American women with an increase in new cases among gay or bisexual men.[2] In 2010, an estimated 26% of new HIV infections occurred in individuals between 13 and 24 years of age, although this age group only comprises approximately 16% of the total US population.[3] With the age of infection becoming younger, it is important that health care providers understand the pathophysiology of HIV, recognize medications that halt the viral replication process, and identify comorbidities that occur in this population. Only through understanding these elements can health care providers improve outcomes, and contribute to the patient's overall quality of life.

Disclosure Statement: The author has no affiliations with or involvement in any organization or entity with any financial interest or nonfinancial interest.
Vanderbilt University School of Nursing, 461 21st Avenue South, Nashville, TN 37240, USA
E-mail address: courtney.j.young@vanderbilt.edu

nursing.theclinics.com

HUMAN IMMUNODEFICIENCY VIRUS PATHOPHYSIOLOGY

The HIV life cycle is complex, and includes binding and entry, reverse transcription, integration, synthesis of viral proteins, and budding (**Fig. 1**). The life cycle begins with the binding of the HIV virion to the glycoproteins 120 and 41, which bind to CD4$^+$ cell receptors and coreceptors of a susceptible cell. Glycoproteins 41 and 120 of the HIV virus interact with CD4$^+$ and CCR5 coreceptors to initiate fusion between the viral envelope and plasma membrane to facilitate entry of the core of the virus into the cytoplasm. Viral RNA is released into the cytoplasm after the core is uncoated, leading to reverse transcription in which the RNA is then converted to DNA provirus. Integration into the host cell's DNA occurs once the provirus migrates into nucleus. At this point in the life cycle, the virus may remain latent. If the infected cell is activated, the provirus is then transcribed and translated into viral protein precursors that are modified by proteases into smaller proteins that assemble the viral RNA into new mature virions that bud from the cell. Each phase of the cycle can be blocked to reduce the number of cell's infected because of viral replication.

ANTIRETROVIRAL THERAPY

There are five antiretroviral therapy (ART) drug classes: (1) nucleotide reverse-transcriptase inhibitors (NRTIs), (2) nonnucleotide reverse-transcriptase inhibitors (NNRTIs), (3) protease inhibitors (PIs), (4) integrase inhibitors (INSTIs), and (5) entry inhibitors. The drug class name indicates the point at which the drug halts the HIV replication process in the life cycle (**Box 1**).

ART regimens are typically composed of a pair of NRTIs and a third drug class so as to stop the HIV life cycle at two different points in the replication process. According to the US Department of Health and Human Services (DHHS), the goal of ART therapy includes, but is not limited to, the reduction of HIV-related morbidity and mortality and control of HIV replication via viral suppression.[4] Viral suppression is achieved when an individual who is infected with HIV has HIV-1 RNA, or viral load, less than 40 copies per milliliter. Currently, there are 26 individual agents and 11 coformulated combination regimens approved by the US Food and Drug Administration (FDA) for the treatment of HIV. Baseline bloodwork, including resistance testing, should be obtained before initiating therapy.

It is also recommended that all individuals that are HIV-positive be treated with ART despite CD4$^+$ count. Baseline bloodwork should include a complete blood count,

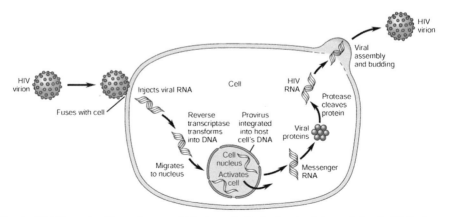

Fig. 1. HIV life cycle. (*From* Copstead LE, Banasik JL. Pathophysiology. St Louis (MO): Saunders/Elsevier; 2007; with permission.)

Box 1	
Antiretroviral classes and action	
Nucleotide reverse-transcriptase inhibitors and nonnucleotide reverse-transcriptase inhibitors	Prevents the production of new viruses by halting the reverse transcriptase of HIV DNA from viral RNA
Protease inhibitors	Blocks HIV enzyme protease to prevent the separation and assembling of HIV polyproteins into individual proteins that produce new virions
Integrase inhibitors	Prevents the integration of HIV DNA into the host cell's DNA
Entry inhibitors	Attaches to the glycoproteins or CCR5 receptors on the surface of T cells preventing HIV from binding to the cell and gaining entry

comprehensive metabolic panel, sexually transmitted infection testing, HIV-1 RNA, $CD4^+$ count/percentage, urinalysis, and hepatitis screening. The prophylaxis against opportunistic infections should be initiated and deemed necessary based on an individual's $CD4^+$ count.

RESISTANCE TESTING

Testing of an individual's HIV-1 RNA is vital to the selection of the appropriate ART regimen. An HIV-1 strain can possibly have mutations present that cause resistance to a particular agent or class of medications resulting in virologic failure of an inaccurately selected regimen. This is important because an estimated one in five individuals are found to have mutations present in their HIV strand on resistance testing.[5] Guidelines recommend genotypic resistance testing before starting or changing an ART regimen.[4,6] A genotype usually tests for resistance among the NRTI, NNRTI, and PI classes. Studies have shown that resistance is highest among the NNRTI class at baseline, which increases the likelihood of NNRTI-based regimens being ineffective in virologic suppression.[7,8]

Integrase inhibitors have a separate INSTI genotype that is not ordered unless an INSTI is being considered for initial therapy and there is cause for concern of possible INSTI resistance. Entry inhibitors have a testing assay (tropism assay) that is used when a CCR5 antagonist is being considered. There are four types of tropism: (1) R5-tropism indicating that the virus exclusively binds to the CCR5 coreceptor, (2) X4-tropism in which the virus exclusively binds to the CXCR4 coreceptor, (3) dual/mixed tropism in which the virus is able to bind to either coreceptor, or (4) mixed-tropism in which there is a mixture of both R5-tropic and X4-tropic viruses. A result of a tropism assay may be listed as dual/mixed because the assay is unable to distinguish between dual-tropism and mixed-tropism. However, a tropism assay is usually needed in more treatment-experienced patients. Only patients with R5-tropic virus are eligible for the consideration of entry inhibitors in their ART regimens only after acquiring mutations and/or experiencing virologic failure with use of previous ART regimens.

UPDATED GUIDELINES FOR FIRST-LINE REGIMENS

As new combination therapies continue to become available, guidelines regarding first-line regimens change to reflect the most effective choices among available regimens in the successful reduction of HIV-1 RNA with minimal side effects. Changes in guidelines regarding ART come from either the DHHS or the International Antiviral Society–USA (IAS-USA). Although the recommendations are similar, there are some differences. In April 2015, DHHS updated its guidelines to exclude NNRTI-based regimens from recommended first-line therapy compared with the July 2015 IAS-USA updated guidelines. Five first-line regimens are recommended as initial therapy by DHHS in these guidelines (**Box 2**).

Recommendations by the IAS-USA panel differ in that it includes (1) the use of the NNRTI efavirenz, to be paired with one of the recommended NRTI pairs; (2) the use of atazanavir/ritonavir as an alternate boosted PI to add to one of the recommended NRTI pairs; and (3) the coformulation of emtricitabine/rilpilvirine/tenofovir, which includes an NNRTI.

DHHS and IAS-USA additionally offer guidelines of alternative regimens that may be used when selecting a regimen based on efficacy of virologic suppression, likelihood of patient adherence, potential toxicity, pill burden, dose frequency, potential drug interactions, treatment of other comorbidities, cost, and resistance testing. The goal of therapy selection is that it is the optimal regimen for viral suppression in the individual, taking into consideration the aforementioned characteristics.

NUCLEOTIDE REVERSE-TRANSCRIPTASE INHIBITORS BACKBONES

Guidelines by the DHHS and IAS-USA recommend that each ART regimen be composed of a pair of NRTIs and a third class that is either a boosted PI or an INSTI, depending on which guideline the clinician uses as a reference. The two common NRTI pairs (emtricitabine/tenofovir and abacavir/lamivudine) are available in fixed-dose once-daily dosing coformulations and assist the clinician in selecting a regimen low in pill burden and potentially cost. There are advantages and disadvantages associated with each coformulation. A third coformulation, lamivudine/zidovudine, is also available for treatment but is used as an alternate NRTI regimen in adults.

Emtricitabine/Tenofovir

Emtricitabine/tenofovir is considered superior in terms of HIV-1 virologic suppression, safety, side effects, and tolerability as demonstrated in studies in which it was compared with lamivudine/zidovudine in addition to the NNRTI efavirenz. It is thereby most recommended for ART regimens in guidelines by DHHS and IAS-USA.[4,9] It can be paired with any of the other classes while taking into consideration the characteristics or needs of the individual being treated in the absence of renal disease.

Box 2
First-line ART regimens recommended as initial therapy by DHHS panel

Abacavir/lamivudine/dolutegravir (only if HLA-B*5701 testing is negative)

Dolutegravir plus emtricitabine/tenofovir

Cobicistat/elvitegravir/emtricitabine/tenofovir (only if creatinine clearance >70 mL/min)

Raltegravir plus emtricitabine/tenofovir

Darunavir/ritanonavir plus emtricitabine/tenofovir

From Panel on Antiretroviral Guidelines for Adults and Adolescents. Guidelines for the use of antiretroviral agents in HIV-1-infected adults and adolescents. Department of Health and Human Services; 2014. Available at: http://aidsinfo.nih.gov/guidelines/html/1/adult-and-adolescent-arv-guidelines/0.

Abacavir/Lamivudine

Abacavir/lamivudine, in conjunction with efavirenz, demonstrated less mitochondrial toxicity, greater mean $CD4^+$ cell count increase, but similar virologic suppression when compared with lamivudine/zidovudine.[10] Additionally, the use of this coformulation with efavirenz demonstrated side effects, such as lipodystrophy, dyslipidemia, and drug discontinuation.[11] DHHS guidelines suggest that this coformulation only be paired with dolutegravir as a recommended first-line regimen versus IAS-USA guidelines, which also recommend pairing it with dolutegravir but lists efavirenz and boosted atazanvir as options.[4]

Emtricitabine/Tenofovir Versus Abacavir/Lamivudine

As the leading two pairs of NRTI backbones, each pair has its own limitations that must be considered when developing an ART regimen. The tenofovir component of the emtricitabine/tenofovir coformulation potentially lends to an increased risk of nephrotoxic effects especially when taken with a PI.[12,13] This adverse effect should be taken into account when considering this coformulation for any individual with renal dysfunction or advanced HIV infection.[14] Individuals with comorbidities that could impact renal function or are prescribed other medications that are potentially nephrotoxic should have their serum creatinine and creatinine clearance cautiously monitored at regular intervals. Abacavir/lamivudine is an option for individuals with renal dysfunction. However, the use of this coformulation is limited in that the individual to be treated must have a negative HLA B*5701 serum test, which would indicate that the individual will not experience a potentially life-threatening hypersensitivity reaction as an adverse effect of this medication and those at high risk or living with cardiovascular disease.[4,6]

Additionally, IAS-USA guidelines note that the abacavir/lamivudine coformulation has demonstrated lower rates of virologic suppression in individuals who have a baseline of greater than 100,000 copies per milliliter of HIV-1 RNA when compared with emtracitabine/tenofovir based on randomized studies of the two backbones being paired with efavirenz or atazanvir/ritonavir.[6,15,16] However, abacavir/lamivudine proves to have less of an impact on bone mineral density and limb fat compared with its NRTI counterpart reducing the risk of fractures.[17]

PREFERRED PROTEASE INHIBITORS

Based on current guidelines by DHHS and IAS-USA, there are three boosted PI agents available for use in combination with the recommended NRTI backbones as first-line or alternative regimens: (1) atazanavir, (2) darunavir, and (3) lopinavir/ritonavir. Ideally, these agents are selected for individuals where the clinician suspects possible low adherence to ART because these medications have a high barrier to resistance. The PIs used in ART regimens are boosted with an additional agent to slow metabolism of the PI, resulting in increased plasma levels. Not only does this reduce dosing frequency, but it also increases the regimen's ability to achieve virologic suppression compared with unboosted PI regimens.

For a period of time, ritonavir was a PI administered in a low dose with other PIs, such as atazanvir or darunavir, to help with the boosting of plasma levels through the inhibition of CYP3A4 liver enzymes. With the coformulation of cobicistat/elvitegravir/emtricitabine/tenofovir came the introduction of a new CYP3A4 inhibitor that could also be used to boost PIs. Currently, there are several boosted PI-based therapy choices that may be used as first-line therapy or alternative options (**Box 3**).[4,6]

Box 3
PI-based therapy choices

Atazanavir/ritonavir

Atazanavir/cobicistat (once-daily fixed coformulation)

Darunavir/ritonavir

Darunavir/cobicistat (once-daily fixed coformulation)

Lopinavir/ritonavir

When considering boosted PIs as a third agent, it is important to consider such characteristics as pill burden, virologic suppression, safety, tolerability, and side effects to decrease the likelihood of nonadherence to the ART regimen.

Protease Inhibitors Boosted with Ritonavir

Ritonavir is a PI given in a low dose (100-mg tablet once daily) to help increase, or boost, plasma levels of other PIs. When comparing the efficacy of boosted PIs, similar results of viral suppression of HIV-1 RNA were observed when comparing atazanavir/ritonavir or darunavir/ritonavir with lopinavir/ritonavir when each of the boosted PIs were given with an emtricitabine/tenofovir regimen in individuals with a baseline of greater than 100,000 copies per milliliter, although the atazanavir/ritonavir and darunavir/ritonavir combinations proved superior in those with baselines between 200 and 100,000 copies per milliliter.[18–20] There are several advantages and disadvantages of boosted PIs (**Table 1**).[18–22]

PIs taken in combination with an NRTI pair containing tenofovir for more than 6 months are at greater risk of causing chronic kidney disease.[13] Additionally, individuals whose regimen included a boosted PI and tenofovir are also at increased risk of fractures secondary to osteoporosis.[23]

Protease Inhibitors Boosted with Cobicistat

Recently, cobicistat was approved by the FDA to be used as a boosting agent with PIs (atazanavir and darunavir). Both PIs are now coformulated with cobicistat into a once-daily dosing to be administered with an NRTI-based pair. In comparison with ritonavir, cobicistat demonstrated similar virologic suppression, safety, tolerability, and adverse effects in patients with HIV, including those whose baseline was greater than 100,000 copies per milliliter.[24] Additionally, cobicistat is more selective than ritonavir, has a low induction potential, and has more predictable drug interactions. The use of these new coformulations has been approved by the DHHS and IAS-USA as alternative regimens in the updated version of the guidelines.[4,6]

There are other PIs available for use in ART regimens. However, some of them are no longer recommended for use in initial therapy because of adverse effects. Fosaprenavir/ritonavir has a high pill burden, gastrointestinal intolerance, and elevated lipids.[4,6,25] Saquinavir/ritonavir has high pill burden, PR and QT interval prolongation, gastrointestinal intolerance, and elevated triglyceride levels, which have led to this agent no longer being recommended for use at all.[26]

CHOOSING AMONG INTEGRASE INHIBITORS

To date, there are three integrase inhibitors available for treatment of ART-naive individuals: (1) raltegravir, (2) dolutegravir, and (3) elvitegravir (**Table 2**). All three agents

Table 1
Preferred protease inhibitors

Protease Inhibitors	Advantages	Disadvantages
Atazanavir/ritonavir	Low pill burden Once-daily dosing No PI cross-resistance Decreased gastrointestinal side effect of diarrhea	Increased bilirubin levels (which may be used to prove adherence) Jaundice Nephrolithiasis Cannot be taken with H_2 blockers/proton pump inhibitors
Darunavir/ritonavir	Lowest pill burden of PIs Once-daily dosing No PI cross-resistance No effects on bilirubin Decreased gastric effects Good central nervous system penetration Deemed superior to other three mentioned for these reasons	Changes in total cholesterol and non-high-density lipoprotein cholesterol Decreased triglycerides levels Monitoring necessary if used in patients with sulfa allergy, rash reaction
Lopinavir/ritonavir	Coformulated with boosting agent PI resistance minimal with virologic failure when first PI taken	Greatest effect on changes in lipid levels compared with darunavir/ritonavir and atazanavir/ritonavir More gastrointestinal side effects compared with darunavir/ritonavir and atazanavir/ritonavir More likely to be discontinued because of toxicity Increased risk of myocardial infarction Higher risk of virologic failure

are a part of one of the five ART combinations recommended as first-line therapy by the DHHS and ISA-USA guidelines. When compared with efaverinz, it was observed that raltegravir and elvitagravir demonstrated similar virologic suppression, whereas dolutegravir was found to be superior.[26–28] It was also found that dolutagravir and raltegravir demonstrated similar virologic suppression and increase in $CD4^+$ cell count, although dolutegravir demonstrated a lower virologic failure rate and higher resistance barrier than its counterpart.[29] Use of both medications resulted in a slight increase in creatinine levels but without effects on glomerular filtration rates or causing adverse renal events.[30]

ENTRY INHIBITORS

Maraviroc is the only entry inhibitor approved for use in antiretroviral-naive individuals by the FDA, although it is not included in the guidelines for first-line therapy by the DHHS or IAS-USA. However, IAS-USA does include in its recommendations the use of Maraviroc in treatment-experienced individuals, but it cannot be used if CXCR4 or dual-mixed tropism is present. Maraviroc has demonstrated inferiority in comparison with the NNRTI efaverinz when in combination with the NRTI backbone of lamivudine/zidovudine because of a greater number of virologic failures and adverse events.[31]

Table 2
Integrase inhibitors used in ART regimens

Integrase Inhibitors	Advantages	Disadvantages
Raltegravir	Rapid viral load suppression Low pill burden Can be used in patients with renal impairment Decreased lipid effects Few drug interactions	Twice-daily dosing Low barrier to resistance with possible resistance to NRTIs with virologic failure Increase in lipid changes
Dolutegravir	Once-daily dosing Decreased lipid effects Few drug interactions	Food requirement Small increase in creatinine levels Gastrointestinal intolerance Decrease in bone mineral density Barrier to resistance currently unknown
Elvitegravir	Once-daily dosing in single pill coformulation with NRTI pair and cobicistat Available as elvitegravir/cobicistat coformulation in case of impaired renal function Decreased lipid effects	Drug interactions Low barrier to resistance with possible resistance to NRTIs with virologic failure Not recommended for individuals with creatinine clearance <70 mL/min

TREATMENT IN PREGNANCY

It is recommended that all pregnant women be treated with ART despite CD4$^+$ count or viral load to ensure the prevention of maternal-fetal transmission through virologic suppression of the mother. Additionally, pre-exposure prophylaxis for the fetus is also recommended. When selecting an ART regimen for women of childbearing age, the possibility of pregnancy must be considered especially if there is uncertainty about contraceptive measures. There are a few differences in recommendations for initial therapy for pregnant women versus their nonpregnant counterparts (**Box 4**).

Pregnant women should continue their prescribed ART regimen intrapartum and postpartum.[33] During the intrapartum period, it is recommended that intravenous zidovudine be administered as deemed necessary. Such situations include women where there is concern for adherence, during labor of a woman with an HIV-1 RNA greater than 1000 copies per milliliter, or when the HIV-1 RNA level is not known. According to Connor and coworkers,[35] the use of intravenous zidovudine has decreased mother-to-fetus transmission by 67.5%. Zidovudine should be discontinued from the oral therapy if intravenous zidovudine is initiated while lamivudine is given at 12-hour intervals.

Cesarean section delivery is the preferred method of delivery for virologically suppressed and women who have not achieved virologic suppression less than 1000 copies per milliliter at 39 and 38 weeks gestation, respectively. According to DHHS, zidovudine prophylaxis should be administered to neonates for 6 weeks. For those neonates who test positive or were born to a mother who was not virologically suppressed, full ART regimen is required.[33] Breastfeeding is not recommended in any HIV-infected woman, regardless of virologic suppression, if there is access to clean water and formula to reduce the risk of mother-to-fetus HIV transmission.[4]

TREATMENT IN CHILDREN AND ADOLESCENTS

Infants, children, and adolescents older than 1 year of age that are treatment-naive should have an ART regimen combination that includes dual-nucleoside/NRTI

> **Box 4**
> **Recommendations for initial therapy for pregnant women by DHHS panel**
>
> - A pair of NRTIs and either an NNRTI or boosted PI is the preferred combination of choice.
>
> - Zidovudine is the preferred agent of choice, although women may experience adverse effects that may be problematic in pregnancy.
>
> - NRTIs with the ability to cross the placenta in high levels (emtricitabine, tenofovir, lamivudine, and zidovudine) should be paired and used as an ART regimen.
>
> - The use of a triple NRTI regimen is not recommended.
>
> - Efavirenz should be avoided in pregnant women and women of childbearing age because of its teratogenic effects and could result in congenital anomalies in infants.[32] An exception is for those pregnant women who present to care already in their first trimester and are virologically suppressed.[33]
>
> - Pregnant women on ART that are virally suppressed should continue their current regimen despite the type of agents being used because of risking the loss of viral suppression because of regimen modification.
>
> - The use of PIs has been associated with preterm delivery in pregnant women. However, there is no association between PI use and hospitalizations or infant death.[34]
>
> - Other comorbidities, potential for adherence, adverse effects, and other characteristics should be taken into consideration when selecting a regimen for a pregnant woman.
>
> *From* Panel on treatment of HIV-infected pregnant women and prevention of perinatal transmission. Recommendations for use of antiretroviral drugs in pregnant HIV-1-Infected women for maternal health and Interventions to reduce perinatal HIV transmission in the United States. Available at: http://aidsinfo.nih.gov/contentfiles/lvguidelines/perinatalgl.pdf. Accessed July 1, 2015.

backbone combination with either an NNRTI or PI.[36] The NRTI pair backbone either consists of abacavir or zidovudine plus either lamivudine or emtracitabine depending on the age of the child:

- For infants aged <3 months: zidovudine plus (lamivudine or emtricitabine)
- For children aged ≥3 months: abacavir plus (lamivudine or emtricitabine) or zidovudine plus (lamivudine or emtricitabine)
- For children aged ≥12 years: abacavir plus lamivudine or plus emtricitabine
- For adolescents at Tanner Stage 4 or 5: abacavir plus lamivudine or plus emtricitabine or tenofovir disoproxil fumarate plus lamivudine or plus emtricitabine

The preferred agent chosen as the third class for use in the ART regimen also depends on the age of the child/adolescent (DHHS):

- For neonates/infants aged ≥42 weeks postmenstrual and ≥14 days postnatal and children <3 years: lopinavir/ritonavir
- For children aged 3 years to <6 years: efavirenz or lopinavir/ritonavir
- For children aged ≥6 years: atazanavir/ritonavir or efavirenz or lopinavir/ritonavir

Just as with adults, there are alternative regimens indicated for children older than 1 year of age that should be considered for therapy selection based on the characteristics and potential adherence of the child being treated.

SUMMARY

The ultimate goal of ART is virologic suppression of an individual infected with HIV. It is imperative that highly effective ART regimens are selected using combinations of the best agents available that have proved to be efficacious, cost-effective, safe, tolerable, and with minimal adverse effects. Regimens must be tailored according to the individual's characteristics and preferences. Keeping well-informed about the most current evidence regarding clinical practices and pharmacologic therapy selections contributes to the overall well-being of persons with HIV. Ensuring that individuals with HIV have access to the quality care necessary to reduce morbidity and mortality, to ameliorate HIV-associated complications, and to improve or maintain quality of life is essential to holistic and competent care.

REFERENCES

1. Centers for Disease Control and Prevention. Estimated HIV incidence among adults and adolescents in the United States, 2007–2010. HIV Surveillance Supplemental Report 2012;17(No. 4). Available at: http://www.cdc.gov/hiv/topics/surveillance/resources/reports/#supplemental. Accessed July 1, 2015.
2. Hall HI, Song R, Rhodes P, et al. Estimation of HIV incidence in the United States. JAMA 2008;300(5):520–9.
3. Purcell D, Johnson CH, Lansky A, et al. Estimating the population size of men who have sex with men in the United States to obtain HIV and syphilis rates. Open AIDS J 2012;6(Suppl 1: m6):114–23.
4. Panel on Antiretroviral Guidelines for Adults and Adolescents. Guidelines for the use of antiretroviral agents in HIV-1-infected adults and adolescents. Department of Health and Human Services; 2014. Available at: http://aidsinfo.nih.gov/guidelines/html/1/adult-and-adolescent-arv-guidelines/0. Accessed July 1, 2015.
5. Ocfemia CB, Kim D, Ziebell R, et al. Prevalence and trends of transmitted drug resistance-associated mutations by duration of infection among persons newly diagnosed with HIV-1 infection: 5 states and 3 municipalities, US, 2006 to 2009. Program and Abstracts of the 19th Conference on Retroviruses and Opportunistic Infections. Seattle (WA), March 5–8, 2012. Abstract 730.
6. Günthard HF, Aberg JA, Eron JJ, et al. Antiretroviral treatment of adult HIV infection: 2014 recommendations of the International Antiviral Society-USA panel. JAMA 2014;312:410–25.
7. Borroto-Esoda K, Waters JM, Bae AS, et al. Baseline genotype as a predictor of virological failure to emtricitabine or stavudine in combination with didanosine and efavirenz. AIDS Res Hum Retroviruses 2007;23:988–95.
8. Kuritzkes DR, Lalama CM, Ribaudo HJ, et al. Preexisting resistance to nonnucleoside reverse-transcriptase inhibitors predicts virologic failure of an efavirenz-based regimen in treatment-naïve HIV-1 infected subjects. J Infect Dis 2008;197:867–70.
9. Gallant JE, DeJesus E, Arribas JR, et al. Tenofovir DF, emtricitabine and efavirenz vs. zidovudine, lamivudine, and efavirenz for HIV. N Engl J Med 2006;354:251–60.
10. DeJesus E, Herrera G, Teofilo E, et al. Abacavir versus zidovudine combined with lamivudine and efavirenz, for the treatment of antiretroviral-naive HIV-infected adults. Clin Infect Dis 2004;39:1038–46.
11. Podzamczer D, Ferrer E, Sanchez P, et al. Less lipoatrophy and better lipid profile with abacavir as compared to stavudine: 96-week results of a randomized study. J Acquir Immune Defic Syndr 2007;44:139–47.
12. Mocroft A, Kirk O, Reiss P, et al. Estimated glomerular filtration rate, chronic kidney disease and antiretroviral drug use in HIV-positive patients. AIDS 2010;24:1667–78.

13. Morlat P, Vivot A, Vandenhende MA, et al. Role of traditional risk factors and antiretroviral drugs in the incidence of chronic kidney disease, ANRS CO3 Aquitaine cohort, France, 2004-2012. PLoS One 2013;8:e66223.
14. Gallant JE, Parish MA, Keruly JC, et al. Changes in renal function associated with tenofovir disoproxil fumarate treatment, compared with nucleoside reverse-transcriptase inhibitor treatment. Clin Infect Dis 2005;40:1194–8.
15. Sax P, Tierney C, Collier A, et al. Abacavir-lamivudine versus tenofovir-emtricitabine for initial HIV-1 therapy. N Engl J Med 2009;361:2230–40.
16. Daar ES, Tierney C, Fischl MA, et al. Atazanavir plus ritonavir or efavirenz as part of a 3-drug regimen for initial treatment of HIV-1: a randomized trial. Ann Intern Med 2011;154:445–56.
17. McComsey GA, Kitch D, Daar ES, et al. Bone mineral density and fractures in antiretroviral-naive persons randomized to receive abacavir-lamivudine or tenofovir disoproxil fumarate-emtricitabine along with efavirenz or atazanavir-ritonavir: AIDS Clinical Trials Group A5224s, a substudy of ACTG A5202. J Infect Dis 2011;203:1791–801.
18. Molina JM, Andrade-Villanueva J, Echevarria J, et al. Once-daily atazanavir/ritonavir versus twice-daily lopinavir/ritonavir, each in combination with tenofovir and emtricitabine, for management of antiretroviral-naive HIV-1-infected patients: 48 week efficacy and safety results of the CASTLE study. Lancet 2008; 372:646–55.
19. Ortiz R, Dejesus E, Khanlou H, et al. Efficacy and safety of once-daily darunavir/ritonavir versus lopinavir/ritonavir in treatment-naive HIV-1-infected patients at week 48. AIDS 2008;22:1389–97.
20. Mills AM, Nelson M, Jayaweera D. Once-daily darunavir/ritonavir vs. lopinavir/ritonavir in treatment-naive, HIV-1-infected patients: 96-week analysis. AIDS 2009; 23:1679–88.
21. Lennox JL, Landovitz RJ, Ribaudo HJ, et al. Efficacy and tolerability of 3 nonnucleoside reverse transcriptase inhibitor-sparing antiretroviral regimens for treatment-naïve volunteers infected with HIV-1: a randomized controlled equivalence trial. Ann Intern Med 2014;161:461–71.
22. Worm W, Sabin C, Weber R, et al. Risk of myocardial infarction in patients with HIV infection exposed to specific individual antiretroviral drugs from the 3 major drug classes: the data collection on adverse events on anti-HIV drugs (D: A:D) study. J Infect Dis 2010;201:318–30.
23. Bedimo R, Maalouf NM, Zhang S, et al. Osteoporotic fracture risk associated with cumulative exposure to tenofovir and other antiretroviral agents. AIDS 2012;26: 825–31.
24. Gallant JE, Koenig E, Andrade-Villanueva J, et al. Cobicistat versus ritonavir as a pharmacoenhancer of atazanavir plus emtricitabine/tenofovir disoproxil fumarate in treatment-naïve HIV type 1-infected patients: week 48 results. J Infect Dis 2013;208:32–9.
25. Enron J Jr, Yeni P, Gathe J Jr, et al. The KLEAN study of fosamprenavir-ritonavir versus lopinavir-ritonavir, each in combination with abacavir-lamivudine, for initial treatment of HIV infection over 48 weeks: a randomized non-inferiority trial. Lancet 2006;368:476–82.
26. Walmsley S, Avihingsanon A, Slim J, et al. Gemini: a noninferiority study of saquinavir/ritonavir versus lopinavir/ritonavir as initial HIV-1 therapy in adults. J Acquir Immune Defic Syndr 2009;50:367–74.
27. Sax PE, DeJesus E, Mills A, et al. Co-formulated elvitegravir, cobicistat, emtricitabine, and tenofovir versus co-formulated efavirenz, emtricitabine, and tenofovir

for initial treatment of HIV-1 infection: a randomised, double-blind, phase 3 trial, analysis of results after 48 weeks. Lancet 2012;379:2439–48.

28. Walmsley SL, Antela A, Clumeck N, et al. Dolutegravir plus abacavir-lamivudine for the treatment of HIV-1 infection. N Engl J Med 2013;369:1807–18.

29. Raffi F, Rachlis A, Stellbrink HJ, et al, SPRING-2 Study Group. Once-daily dolutegravir versus raltegravir in antiretroviral-naive adults with HIV-1 infection: 48 week results from the randomised, double-blind, non-inferiority SPRING-2 study. Lancet 2013;381:735–43.

30. Koteff J, Borland J, Chen S, et al. A phase 1 study to evaluate the effect of dolutegravir on renal function via measurement of iohexol and para-aminohippurate clearance in healthy subjects. Br J Clin Pharmacol 2013;75:990–6.

31. Cooper DA, Herra J, Goodrich J, et al. Maraviroc versus efavirenz, both in combination with zidovudine-lamivudine, for the treatment of antiretroviral-naïve subjects with CCR5-tropic HIV-1 infection. J Infect Dis 2010;201:803–13.

32. Brogly SB, Abzug MJ, Watts DH, et al. Birth defects among children born to human immunodeficiency virus-infected women: pediatric AIDS clinical trials protocols 219 and 219C. Pediatr Infect Dis J 2010;29:721–7.

33. Panel on treatment of HIV-infected pregnant women and prevention of perinatal transmission. Recommendations for use of antiretroviral drugs in pregnant HIV-1-Infected women for maternal health and Interventions to reduce perinatal HIV transmission in the United States. Available at: http://aidsinfo.nih.gov/contentfiles/lvguidelines/perinatalgl.pdf. Accessed July 1, 2015.

34. Powis KM, Kitch D, Ogwu A, et al. Increased risk of preterm delivery among HIV-infected women randomized to protease versus nucleoside reverse transcriptase inhibitor-based HAART during pregnancy. J Infect Dis 2011;204:506–14.

35. Connor RI, Sheridan KE, Ceradini D, et al. Change in coreceptor use correlates with disease progression in HIV-1-infected individuals. J Exp Med 1997;185(4):621–8. Available at: http://www.ncbi.nlm.nih.gov/entrez/query.fcgi?cmd=Retrieve&db=PubMed&dopt=Citation&list_uids=9034141.

36. Panel on Antiretroviral Therapy and Medical Management of HIV-Infected Children. Guidelines for the use of antiretroviral agents in pediatric HIV infection. Available at: http://aidsinfo.nih.gov/contentfiles/lvguidelines/pediatricguidelines.pdf. Accessed July1, 2015.

Pharmacologic Strategies for Treatment of Poisonings

Eric Roberts, DNP, FNP-BC, ENP-BC[a],*,
Michael D. Gooch, MSN, ACNP-BC, FNP-BC, ENP-BC[b,c,d,e]

KEYWORDS

- Toxicology • Toxidromes • Drug abuse • Street drugs • Overdoses

KEY POINTS

- Poisoning is the leading cause of injury-related mortality in the United States, with more than 40,000 deaths annually.
- Toxicologic emergencies range from intentional to accidental overdoses and include substances both legal and illegal.
- Toxidromes assist the clinician in narrowing the differential diagnosis through an understanding of global symptoms common to categorical poisonings.
- Pharmacologic management may be determined by understanding the toxidrome categories.

INTRODUCTION

Poisoning is the leading cause of injury-related mortality in the United States, with more than 40,000 deaths annually.[1] To ensure optimal patient outcomes in poisoning situations, nurses must have foundational knowledge of overdoses and how to effectively intervene. Prescribed drugs, over-the-counter drugs, and illegal drugs can all contribute to intentional or unintentional overdoses to various extent and mandate thorough consideration. From 2008 to 2011, an estimated 1.1 million patients annually went to emergency departments for drug poisonings at a rate of 35.4 per 10,000 persons.[2] Nearly one-quarter (24.5%) of these visits resulted in hospital admission.

Trends suggest the need for a heightened knowledge and ability to manage toxicologic emergencies. Between 2004 and 2009 there was a 98.4% increase in

Disclosures: None.
[a] Loyola University Chicago, 2160 South First Avenue, Marcella Niehoff School of Nursing Building, Room 4500, Maywood, IL 60153, USA; [b] Vanderbilt University School of Nursing, Nashville, TN, USA; [c] Middle Tennessee School of Anesthesia, Madison, TN, USA; [d] Vanderbilt University Medical Center - LifeFlight, Nashville, TN, USA; [e] TeamHealth at Maury Regional Medical Center, Columbia, TN, USA
* Corresponding author.
E-mail address: robertsdnp@gmail.com

nonmedical use of pharmaceuticals. During this same period, there was an 82.9% increase in emergency department visits involving adverse reactions to drugs.[3] Opioids were the most frequent class of drugs that prompted emergency department visits. Use of nonmedical opioids accounted for about 50% of these visits. Illicit drug use is also on the rise with an 8.3% increase in overall illicit drug use from 2002 to 2013.[3] Although cocaine use has declined, there has been an increased use of methamphetamines. Another recent trend in the United States is the increase of drug use seen in persons in their fifties and sixties. This is an important consideration because the pharmacokinetics and pharmacodynamics are quite different in this age group as opposed to younger adult populations.

The complexity of the issue is enhanced when one considers the increasing number and types of drugs along with the diversity of populations using these drugs. To provide optimal care in cases of toxic ingestions, it is essential that health care providers develop knowledge and skills in not only recognizing common presentations, but also to intervene with effective treatment modalities. Although there are numerous agents that can cause toxicities, the scope of this article focuses on more commonly encountered substances and their appropriate antidotes. Toxidromes, describing classical findings of physical examination from a given overdose, are discussed to guide the health care provider in recognizing common diagnoses and treatments of toxicologic emergencies.[4]

TOXIDROMES

Toxidromes are classifications of ingestions based on common presentations and can assist the health care provider in identification of unknown ingestions and focus initial treatment regimens. Caution must be taken when considering toxidromes, however, because comorbidities, ingestion of multiple drugs, and concurrent drug therapies may alter an individual presentation.[4] **Table 1** outlines common toxidromes including anticholinergic, cholinergic, opioid, and sympathomimetic presentations. In general,

Table 1
Common toxidromes

Toxidrome	Evaluation Finding	Drug Example	Treatment
Sympathomimetic	Tachycardia, hypertension, tachypnea, agitation, diaphoresis	Amphetamines, cocaine, PCP, ecstasy, methamphetamine, Ritalin	Intravenous fluids, benzodiazepines, airway support, cardiac monitoring
Anticholinergic	Anhidrosis, mydriasis, flushing, hyperthermia, delirium, seizure, urinary retention, thirst	Antihistamines, antispasmotics, antiparkinson, antipsychotic, antidepressant, phenothiazines	Intravenous fluids, benzodiazepines, antipyretics, physostigmine
Cholinergic	DUMBBELSS	Organophosphates, carbamates, mushrooms, nicotine, pilocarpine	Atropine, pralidoxime
Opioid	Hypoventilation, central nervous system depression, meiosis, hypotension	Hydrocodone, hydromorphone, oxycodone, methadone, fentanyl	Naloxone

vital signs, mental status, pupil size, skin, and mucous membranes are the most useful in determining a specific toxidrome.[5]

Sympathomimetic

Increased activity of alpha and beta receptors typically found in the skin, eyes, heart, lungs, gastrointestinal (GI) tract, exocrine glands, and some neural tracts of the central nervous system are responsible for symptoms found in the sympathomimetic toxidrome.[4] Stimulation at these sites produces tachycardia, hypertension, tachypnea, agitation, and diaphoresis. Amphetamines, cocaine, PCP, ecstasy, methamphetamine, caffeine, cold remedies, pseudoephedrine, methylphenidate (Ritalin), and phencyclidine are examples of sympathomimetic agents. General management includes the use of intravenous (IV) fluids, benzodiazepines, and airway and cardiac monitoring.[6]

Anticholinergic (Antimuscarinic)

Anticholinergic agents are primarily associated with the parasympathetic nervous system, which innervates the eye, heart, respiratory system, skin, GI tract, bladder, and sweat glands.[4] Symptoms of this toxidrome may be recalled using the saying: "dry as a bone, blind as a bat, red as a beet, hot as a hades, mad as a hatter, and sick like a seizure." These correspond with anhidrosis, mydriasis, flushing, hyperthermia, delirium, and seizure, respectively.[4] These patients may also show signs of tachycardia, tachypnea, hypertension, seizures, decreased bowel sounds, thirst, and urinary retention.[6] Drugs found in this class include antihistamines, antispasmotics, atropine, antiparkinson drugs, antipsychotics, antidepressants, and phenothiazines.[7] A general approach to the patient with these exposures involves maintaining an airway, correct hypotension with IV fluid boluses, benzodiazepines, antipyretics, and physostigmine for seizures or resistant dysrhythmias.[6]

Cholinergic

As expected, the cholinergic toxidrome is the opposite presentation of the anticholinergic toxidrome. Cholinergic agents activate muscarinic acetylcholine receptors. A pneumonic used to recall symptoms of cholinergic crisis is DUMBBELLS, which stands for defecation, urination, miosis, bradycardia, bronchospasm, emesis, lacrimation, secretions, and seizures.[6] Organophosphates (nerve gas, insecticides, and pesticides), carbamates, mushrooms, nicotine, and pilocarpine are drugs that may produce this affect.[6] Atropine is the initial drug of choice to treat a cholinergic crisis. In fact, tachycardia is not a contraindication to atropine administration because drying of the respiratory tract and resolution of bronchospasm are priorities.[4] Additionally, if organophosphates are the causative agent, IV pralidoxime should be administered.[6]

Opioid

Opiates include naturally occurring agents, such as morphine and codeine. There are also synthetic opioids, such as hydrocodone, hydromorphone, oxycodone, methadone, and fentanyl.[4] These bind to opioid receptors (mu, kappa, and delta). Each drug affects receptors in slightly different profiles and therefore has potentially different pathologies.[4] In general, these patients experience hypoventilation, central nervous system depression, meiosis, and hypotension.[6] Specifically, tramadol, meperidine, and fentanyl have serotonergic properties and may lead to a serotonin syndrome when combined with other serotonin agonists.[4] Supportive care includes providing oxygenation and airway support when necessary. Opioid poisoning may be reversed with naloxone administered 0.4 to 2 mg every 2 to 3 minutes as needed by IV, subcutaneous, intramuscular, intranasal, and endotracheal routes.[6] Caution must be given when using naloxone to reverse opioid toxicity for two reasons. First, administration may precipitate profound withdrawal symptoms, such as agitation, vomiting, diarrhea, diaphoresis, and yawning.[4] Additionally, because naloxone has a shorter half-life than most opioids, sedation may reoccur. Patients should be observed after naloxone reversal for at least 4 hours for this reason.[4] When the patient experiences recurrent episodes of sedation, a continuous IV infusion of naloxone at a rate of 0.04 to 0.16 mg/kg/h may be indicated.[8]

COMMON PHARMACOLOGIC AGENTS

When considering the risk for toxicity, there are several important factors that must be considered. Among these are the dose of the medication that was ingested and the pharmacokinetics of the substance including drug absorption and elimination. Other factors that deserve attention include the age of the person, and the baseline health at the time of ingestion. These elements come together and greatly impact the outcome of the event.

Certain drugs are associated with toxicities in greater frequency because of their accessibility, rate at which they are prescribed, and presence of narrow therapeutic indices. Included in this review are drugs that are routinely encountered in toxic emergencies. Epidemiologic data, keys for recognition, and interventions are discussed.

Acetaminophen

Acetaminophen is widely available in stand-alone preparations and combination drugs in over-the-counter and prescriptive formulations. An estimated 43 million adults in the United States are taking some form of acetaminophen.[9] This large exposure provides an opportunity for intentional and unintentional overdoses. There is a common misperception among many that drugs purchased over the counter are benign, and do not pose a health risk. In reality, acetaminophen is the most common cause of acute liver failure in the United States, and is responsible for 26,000 hospitalizations with more than 450 deaths annually.[10,11] The liver is responsible for normal excretion of acetaminophen. There is danger when the liver becomes overwhelmed by high doses. Instead of breaking down and excreting the metabolite, it begins to accumulate within the liver cells and destroys them.[12] This creates profound metabolic disturbances because of the resulting loss of liver function that include hypophosphatemia, hypoglycemia, and metabolic acidosis. For adults, a single dose of 10 to 15 g may cause this hepatic necrosis.[13] What is difficult is that damage to the liver only becomes apparent 24 to 48 hours after ingestion and follows a predictable pattern of injury (**Table 2**).[12]

With all ingestions, particularly with acetaminophen ingestions, establishing the time of ingestion is crucial in determining appropriate treatment modalities. Pairing this information with a serum acetaminophen concentration helps determine toxicity for a given ingestion. These values are plotted against a Rumack-Matthew nomogram graph to predict hepatotoxicity and determine the need for treatment.[14] This means that there is not a static number that correlates with toxicity. Rather, the nomogram graph helps one understand a toxic level, as the amount ingested is plotted against time for a specific incident. After plotting these data on a graph, if the serum acetaminophen level is determined to be below the nomogram hepatotoxicity line at 4 hours after ingestion, the patient can safely be discharged. The 4-hour time marker is also important, because if the patient receives medical attention within this time, oral activated charcoal may be administered to prevent further absorption.

Table 2
Symptoms of liver damage postingestion of acetaminophen

Phase	Time Interval Postingestion	Symptoms
1	0–24 h	Malaise, diaphoresis, mild gastric upset
2	24–48 h	Right upper quadrant pain, rise in liver function tests (AST most sensitive), prolonged partial thromboplastin time, and hepatomegaly
3	72–96 h	Massive hepatic dysfunction, jaundice, hypoglycemia, nausea/vomiting, right upper quadrant pain, coagulopathy, and metabolic acidosis
4	4 d to 2 wk	Resolution of liver function tests or death

Abbreviation: AST, aspartate aminotransferase test.
Adapted from Chun L, Tong M, Busuttel R, et al. Acetaminophen hepatotoxicity and liver failure. J Clin Gastroenterol 2009;43:343; with permission.

If the nomogram plot suggests a toxic level, meaning the plot on the graph is above the hepatotoxic line, *N*-acetylcysteine should be administered. This antidote for acetaminophen poisoning should be infused intravenously at 300 mg/kg over 21 hours. Because time is critical, it should also be administered if a serum acetaminophen level will not be available within 8 hours and the total amount ingested is suspected to be at least 7.5 g in an adult or 140 mg/kg in a child.[15] Oral dosing for *N*-acetylcysteine is also available when IV access is not possible.

Salicylates

Salicylate poisonings are associated with high mortality rates unless treated early and aggressively.[16] Salicylates are commonly found in combination drugs making them a source for unintentional overdose. Patients may supplement their combination drugs with additional salicylates not understanding the danger. Salicylates are found in immediate-release formula, which is readily absorbed in the stomach and GI tract within 1 hour. Enteric coated preparations have delayed effect because they pass through the stomach and are absorbed in the small intestine.[17] Absorption can also be prolonged as a result of a large quantity of pills becoming concentrated, forming complex masses in the intestine.[18] The serum half-life of salicylates is typically 2 to 4 hours in low doses and as much as 12 hours when taken in higher doses.[19]

Signs and symptoms are dose and time dependent. Early signs include nausea and vomiting related to GI tract irritation. This may lead to volume depletion, which potentiates late findings. At salicylate levels of 20 to 45 mg/dL or higher the patient experiences tinnitus, hearing loss, or muffling of sounds.[17] The respiratory center becomes stimulated, which leads to hyperventilation and respiratory alkalosis.[20] To compensate, metabolic acidosis and hyperthermia develops.[17] With acidosis, salicylate molecules cross the blood-brain barrier resulting in confusion, delirium, seizures, confusion, or coma.[17] Noncardiac pulmonary edema is a characteristic late sign of progressive salicylate toxicity resulting from increased permeability of the pulmonary vessels.[21]

Treatment of salicylate toxicity is focused on airway management to control hyperventilation, IV fluid replacement to minimize dehydration, correction of electrolyte imbalance, and alkalization of the blood. Alkalization causes salicylate to ionize, which prevents it from crossing of the blood-brain barrier and promotes urinary excretion.[17,18,21] This is accomplished by infusing D5W IV at a rate of 150 to 200 mL/h and adding two to three ampules of sodium bicarbonate to each liter of IV fluid.[18]

Arterial blood gasses and urinary pH should be monitored frequently (often, every 2 hours) along with monitoring for hypoglycemia and hypokalemia.[22] Administration of IV potassium may be required should hypokalemia occur during the alkalization. Hemodialysis should be initiated in acute poisoning when salicylate levels exceed 90 mg/dL.[21]

β-Blockers and Calcium Channel Blockers

β-Blockers and calcium channel blockers are often used to manage hypertension, cardiac arrhythmias, and heart failure. The chronotropic and dromotropic effects of these medications are therapeutic and lifesaving, but in toxic doses they are severe and life threatening. Patients may experience severe bradycardia, dysrhythmias, hypotension, and respiratory distress when taken in higher doses. Conventional management of these toxic scenarios may include the administration of IV fluids, initiation of a vasopressor or inotropic infusion, and overdrive pacing.[23–26]

To ameliorate cardiotoxicity that can occur in β-blocker and calcium channel blocker overdose, targeted pharmacologic treatment may also be used. Glucagon, a pancreatic hormone, is sometimes used for its positive inotropic and chronotropic effects if traditional treatments are not successful.[23,25,26] Most often, glucagon is given as an IV bolus and followed by an infusion. To offset the common side effect of vomiting with administration, glucagon should be administered slowly and following premedication with an antiemetic.[23,26] Patients suffering from a calcium channel blocker overdose may benefit from the IV administration of calcium. Increasing the serum calcium concentration may help overcome the calcium blockade in the cardiac cells, therefore improving contractility and heart rate.[23,25,26]

Two newer treatment modalities include the administration of emulsion lipids and high-dose insulin therapy. IV lipid emulsion therapy has been shown to reduce the toxic effects of lipophilic medications including some β and calcium channel blockers. The lipid emulsion creates a lipid sink, which attracts and pulls lipophilic medications into the vascular bed and frees up the cardiac cells to be more active. The fatty acids from the lipids are also an excellent source of energy and improve calcium channel function in the cardiac cells.[23–25,27]

High-dose insulin therapy with dextrose, also known as hyperinsulinemia/euglycemia, may also prove beneficial in patients with cardiotoxicity. Insulin has positive inotropic effects, similar to glucagon, and also increases cellular uptake of glucose to improve energy production.[23–26] Dextrose should be administered concurrently to prevent hypoglycemia unless the patient is already hyperglycemic. Potassium and glucose levels should be monitored frequently during administration of high-dose insulin therapy.[23,26] When initiating insulin infusion, glucose levels should be monitored every 10 minutes. Once stable, they should be checked every 30 to 60 minutes.[26] Potassium levels should initially be checked hourly and then every 6 hours once stable.[26] A case of metoprolol overdose and successful outcome is presented in **Box 1**.

Toxic Alcohols

Although the most commonly ingested alcohol is ethanol, occasionally a patient is encountered who has consumed another form of alcohol, such as antifreeze or wood alcohol. Toxic alcohol ingestions may be accidental (frequently the case in pediatric populations), but may also be seen as a suicide attempt or as a substitute to satisfy a craving when ethanol is not available.[28,29] Isopropyl alcohol, commonly found in rubbing alcohol, perfumes, some window cleaners, and some solvents, is usually nontoxic.[23] It is more potent than ethanol and results in intoxication, but is usually

---

Box 1
Actual case of metoprolol overdose

A 59-year-old man intentionally overdosed on more than 7.5 g of metoprolol. He presented in severe cardiogenic shock that progressed to cardiac arrest. Conventional efforts were not successful despite vasopressors, inotropes, and glucagon. High-dose insulin therapy and intravenous lipid emulsion therapies were initiated and a pulse was regained. Efforts were continued for 36 hours as he was stabilized. He was successfully treated and recovered.

Although lipid emulsion therapy and high-dose insulin are not initial therapies, they have both proved effective alternatives for patients suffering hemodynamic instability from β-blocker or calcium channel blocker toxicity who are not responding to conventional treatments.

Adapted from Barton C, Johnson N, Mah N, et al. Successful treatment of a massive metoprolol overdose using intravenous lipid emulsion and hyperinsulinemia/euglycemia therapy. Pharmacotherapy 2015;35(5):e57; with permission.

---

nonfatal. It is metabolized to acetone, but does not result in acidosis and management is only supportive unless there was coingestion with another toxic substance.[23]

Ethylene glycol, a common ingredient in antifreeze, deicing solutions, solvents, and some brake fluids, is often toxic if more than 1 mL/kg is ingested.[23] As with ethanol, ethylene glycol is rapidly metabolized and the patient exhibits signs of intoxication within 1 hour of consumption. Metabolites glycolic acid and calcium oxalate lead to a significant metabolic acidosis and renal failure.[23,28,29] Signs of intoxication including altered mental status, tachycardia, hypertension, and Kussmaul respirations occur in response to the impending acidosis. If untreated, seizures, coma, and death soon follow.[23,28,29]

Methanol, or wood alcohol, is often found in solvents, solid fuels, and as a fuel additive. Ingestions in amounts greater than 0.5 mL/kg are usually lethal in most patients.[23] As with ethylene glycol it can lead to signs of intoxication within 1 hour of ingestion, but may cause GI distress. Methanol is metabolized to formaldehyde then to formic acid, resulting in a metabolic gap acidosis. Papilledema and blindness are common complications.[23,28,29]

Definitive management for significant methanol and ethylene glycol ingestions is often best accomplished with hemodialysis to remove the toxins and manage the acidosis.[23,28–30] Until this is performed attention should be focused on securing the patient's airway. In many situations the patient needs IV fluids to maintain tissue perfusion, and if identified, an antidote should be administered.[29] Decontamination of GI tract, functionally removing the toxin generally with activated charcoal, is ineffective and is not recommended.[28]

There are two approaches that are effective in limiting this toxicity which work by inhibiting the metabolism of toxic alcohols. These interventions can also impede the onset of acidosis. First, fomepizole (Antizole) should be administered to inhibit alcohol dehydrogenase, the enzyme in the liver that metabolizes alcohols, until dialysis is accomplished.[23,28–30] Because it is the metabolites of the alcohols that are lethal, and not the alcohols themselves, the administration of fomepizole may prevent the need for hemodialysis in some patients, particularly those without signs of renal or optical injury.[29,30] The second approach involves the administration of ethanol, which is not approved by the Food and Drug Administration, by mouth or intravenously to delay the onset of the toxicity if fomepizole is not available. Alcohol dehydrogenase has a higher affinity to ethanol than other alcohols and selectively metabolizes ethanol first if it is present in higher quantities.[23,28–30] When this is used, a serum ethanol level must be maintained until the toxic alcohol is fully dialyzed.

ILLICIT SUBSTANCES

Over the last decade there has been an increase in the abuse of new illicit drugs. The popularity of these drugs has been fueled by their availability and multiple online sources stating they are safe.[31] Many can be obtained from the Internet, in tobacco shops, or in convenience stores. They are sold under various names without their ingredients listed, and are often labeled "not for human consumption."[31–34] The Drug Enforcement Agency and similar agencies around the world have worked diligently to curtail their availability and abuse. Although most of these drugs or their active ingredients have been listed as Schedule I controlled substances making them illegal in the United States, this has done little to deter the abuse.[31–34] As with many drugs of abuse, these newer designer drugs are highly addictive. As a result, users develop a tolerance and require increasing dosages each time to get the desired effect. This often leads to withdrawal symptoms with abstinence.[31,32] These drugs are often combined with other substances when they are made, exposing users to other harmful substances of which they may be unaware. It is also very common for users to ingest more than one type of drug at a time. This exacerbates intoxication symptoms, and contributes to a myriad of complications that may ensue.

Bath Salts

Bath salts are synthetic amphetamine-like substances that when abused are usually snorted, smoked, or injected. The new trend is to vap them in electronic cigarettes. They are often sold under the names Ivory Wave, Vanilla Sky, Zoom, and Bliss.[31–33,35] The active ingredients often include either 3,4-methylenedioxypyrovalerone or 4-methylmethcathinone (mephedrone), which mimic cathinone, a naturally occurring psychostimulant found in the khat plant.[31–34] Each designer drug has its own unique chemical formulation that changes frequently to avoid legal prosecution and detection by drug tests.[32] Routine drug screens do not detect bath salt compounds. There are some commercial drug detection kits available, but these are rarely available at the bedside and treatment should not be delayed.[32,35]

Euphoria, enhanced sexual arousal, increased alertness, and decreased inhibitions are the effects most users hope to achieve with bath salts abuse.[33,34] Clinical manifestations of bath salt abuse can consist of physical and behavioral effects related to the agonist and antagonist effects on the release and reuptake of three neurotransmitters: (1) dopamine, (2) serotonin, and (3) norepinephrine.[33] Tachycardia, hypertension, hyperthermia, mydriasis, tremors, and cardiac dysrhythmias are common physical symptoms.[31,32,35] Severe complications can include seizures, rhabdomyolysis, renal failure, myocardial infarction, stroke, and death.[31,32,35] The behavioral symptoms, just like the physical symptoms, are related to the overstimulation of the sympathetic nervous system. The patients are often anxious, agitated, and/or aggressive. They may experience hallucinations and even become paranoid, psychotic, suicidal, or violent.[31–33,35]

Initial interventions usually center on ensuring the safety of the health care provider and medical staff. Patients require cooling measures if they are hyperthermic and hydration with IV fluids to prevent renal injury and restore vascular volume.[32,35] Benzodiazepines, such as midazolam (Versed), are the medications of choice to control the hyperexcitability, hypertension, and seizures, if needed.[31–33,35,36] Patients may require an intramuscular or IV bolus or continuous infusions depending on the severity of their intoxication. If further sedation or control of a psychosis is needed then an antipsychotic medication may need to be administered.[32,35,36]

Synthetic Cannabinoids

Spice and K2 are herbal incense or potpourri that have been treated with chemicals to stimulate central and peripheral cannabinoid receptors and produce the typical effects of delta-9-tetrahydrocannabinol (THC) for the user.[34,37] Similar to bath salts, these synthetic cannabinoids (SCBs) have been marketed as safe and a legal version of marijuana. Because they are synthetic, they are not detected through a routine drug screen.[37] Because they are not regulated, there is no consistency on the amount of the chemical or other chemicals in each consumable package. This increases the risk for toxicity. SCBs are most often smoked, but can be ingested. These chemicals are more potent than THC, the active ingredient in marijuana. They have a stronger affinity to the cannabinoid and opioid receptors and therefore produce a stronger and more prolonged response.[34,37] The SCBs can have manifestations similar to those of bath salts, along with GI distress.[34,37] A lesser known effect of THC is its ability to increase sympathetic activity and inhibit parasympathetic activity, which explains why SCBs can cause tachycardia, hypertension, and other stimulating effects.[7] Management of an exposure often only requires supportive care, but if the patient is experiencing significant side effects related to the sympathomimetic effects, then management of intoxication is indicated.[37]

Molly's Plant Food

Molly's Plant Food, in which mephedrone is the active ingredient, uses this common household term to denote an illicit substance and is sold in tobacco shops and on the Internet. In this preparation, it has an action almost identical to 3,4-methylenedioxy-methamphetamine (MDMA) or ecstasy. Ecstasy has been around for several decades and is an amphetamine-like compound with hallucinogenic properties.[38,39] MDMA was once mostly seen as a "rave drug," but it is now more widely used.[39] It is mostly taken orally and increases serotonin levels with lesser effects on dopamine levels. This elevates mood and energy, and also increases the release of oxytocin, cortisol, and antidiuretic hormone.[38] This increase in oxytocin influences one's desire to be with someone and close to others and has earned it the nicknames "love drug" and "hug drug."

Because the desire to be with others is heightened, MDMA is associated with risky sexual activities, transmission of sexually transmitted infections, and even sexual assaults.[38,39] As with the previously mentioned drugs, this increased release in neurotransmitters causes adrenergic effects. Severe hyperthermia and rhabdomyolysis has resulted from serotonin syndrome in some users.[38,39] Hyponatremia and seizures have occurred related to excess release of antidiuretic hormone and the increased reabsorption of water in the kidneys, but is also related to the increased intake of water by some in an effort to avoid overheating and dehydration because MDMA is known to blunt the thirst response.[38,39] As with other sympathomimetics, patients experiencing hyperactivity, hypertension, hyperthermia, and seizures should be managed with cooling measures and benzodiazepines.[38]

SUMMARY

Interventions for optimal outcomes for patients with presumed ingestions are contingent on rapid and accurate identification of the agent, time since ingestion, and current clinical manifestations. Such factors as age and baseline health state also impact the treatments and outcomes for these patients. For the intervention to be efficient, health care providers must have the knowledge to identify the agent, and use approved and appropriate interventions based on patient presentation. Dose, time from ingestion, absorption, and elimination are important when considering risk for toxicity and the required pharmacologic support. There is commonality in providing supportive care to patients, but treatment must be individualized based on underlying pathology, mechanism of action, individual risk, and antidotes specific to provoking agents to ensure the most efficacious patient outcomes possible.

This is an ongoing problem in the health care system, which is further enhanced by the advent of a variety of drugs that are abused, along with clandestine marketing and lack of full disclosure of the contents. It is essential that health care workers have current and accurate knowledge, not only to optimize interventions in situations of abuse, but also for patient and community education. Because legislation has not been completely effective in addressing the problems of access and abuse, an appropriate strategy is to provide information to the public for appropriate intervention, and for patient and community education, current and accurate knowledge of these agents, along with interventions, and availability. Because street drugs change frequently and people often alter illicit use patterns of legal pharmaceuticals, it is important to continually review toxicology trends at the local geographic and national levels.

REFERENCES

1. Warner M, Chen LH, Makuc DM, et al. Drug poisoning deaths in the United States, 1980–2008. NCHS data brief, no 81. Hyattsville (MD): National Center for Health Statistics; 2011.
2. Albert M, McCaig L, Uddin S. Emergency department visits for drug poisoning: United States 2008, 2011. Hyattsville (MD): Centers for Disease Control and Prevention; 2015. NCHS Data Brief, No. 196.
3. National Institute of Health, National Institute on Drug Abuse. Drug Facts: Drug Related Emergency Room Visits. 2011. Available at: http://www.drugabuse.gov/publications/drugfacts/drug-related-hospital-emergency-room-visits. Accessed August 29, 2015.
4. Holstege C, Borek H. Toxidromes. Crit Care Clin 2012;28:479–98.
5. Gresham C, Wilbeck J. Toxicology in the emergency department: a review for the advance practice nurse. Adv Emerg Nurs J 2011;34(1):43–54.
6. Singer A, Burstein J, Schiavone F. Emergency medicine pearls. 2nd edition. Philadelphia: F.A. Davis Company; 2001.
7. Clark BC, Georgekutty J, Berul CI. Myocardial ischemia secondary to synthetic cannabinoid (K2) use in pediatric patients. J Pediatr 2015;167(3):757–61.e1.
8. Keim S, Gomella L, editors. Emergency medicine on call. New York: Lange Medical Books/McGraw-Hill; 2004.
9. Blieden M, Paramore LC, Shah D, et al. A perspective on the epidemiology of acetaminophen exposure and toxicity in the United States. Expert Rev Clin Pharmacol 2014;7(3):341–8.
10. Nourjah P, Ahmad SR, Karwoski C, et al. Estimates of acetaminophen (Paracetamol)-associated overdoses in the United States. Pharmacoepidemiol Drug Saf 2006;15:398–405.
11. Larson AM, Polson J, Fontana RJ, et al. Acetaminophen induced acute liver failure: results of a United States multicenter, prospective study. Hepatology 2005;42:1364–72.

12. Chun L, Tong M, Busuttel R, et al. Acetaminophen hepatotoxicity and liver failure. J Clin Gastroenterol 2009;43:342–9.
13. Budnitz D, Lovegrove M, Crosby A. Emergency department visits for overdoses of acetaminophen-containing products. Am J Prev Med 2011;40(6): 585–92.
14. Larson AM. Acetaminophen hepatotoxicity. Clin Liver Dis 2007;11:525–48.
15. Smilkstein MJ, Knapp GL, Kulig KW, et al. Efficacy of oral N-acetylcysteine in the treatment of acetaminophen overdose. Analysis of the national multicenter study (1976 to 1985). N Engl J Med 1988;319(24):1557–62.
16. Anderson R, Potts D, Gabow P, et al. Unrecognized adult salicylate intoxication. Ann Intern Med 1976;85(6):745–8.
17. Flomenbaum N, Goldfrank L, Hoffman R, et al. Goldfrank's toxicologic emergencies. 8th edition. New York: McGraw-Hill; 2007. p. 550–64.
18. O'Malley G. Emergency department management of the salicylate poisoned patient. Emerg Med Clin North Am 2007;25:333–46.
19. Chyka P, Erdman A, Christianson G, et al. Salicylate poisoning: an evidence based consensus guideline for out of hospital management. Clin Toxicol (Phila) 2007;45(2):95–131.
20. Olsen K, editor. Poisoning & drug overdose. 4th edition. East Norwalk (CT): Appleton & Lange; 2004. p. 331–3.
21. Dart R. Medical toxicology. 3rd edition. Philadelphia: Lippincott Williams & Wilkins; 2004. p. 739–49.
22. Phillips M. Salicylate poisoning. Adv Emerg Nurs J 2008;30(1):75–86.
23. Murray L, Daly F, Little M, et al. Toxicology handbook. 2nd edition. Sydney (Australia): Churchill Livingstone; 2011.
24. Barton C, Johnson N, Mah N, et al. Successful treatment of a massive metoprolol overdose using intravenous lipid emulsion and hyperinsulinemia/euglycemia therapy. Pharmacotherapy 2015;35(5):e56–60.
25. Doepker B, Healy W, Cortez E, et al. High-dose insulin and intravenous lipid emulsion therapy for cardiogenic shock induced by intentional calcium-channel blocker and beta-blocker overdose: a case series. J Emerg Med 2014;46(4):486–90.
26. Engebretsen KM, Kaczmarek KM, Morgan J, et al. High-dose insulin therapy in beta-blocker and calcium channel-blocker poisoning. Clin Toxicol (Phila) 2011; 49(4):277–83.
27. Schultz A, Lewis T, Reed B, et al. That's a phat antidote. Intravenous fat emulsions and toxicological emergencies. Adv Emerg Nurs J 2015;37(3):162–75.
28. McMahon D, Winstead S, Weant K. Toxic alcohol ingestions focus on ethylene glycol and methanol. Adv Emerg Nurs J 2009;31(3):206–13.
29. Rietjens S, de Lange D, Meulenbelt J. Ethylene glycol or methanol intoxication: which antidote should be used, fomepizole or ethanol? Neth J Med 2014;72(2): 73–9.
30. Mégarbane B, Borron SW, Baud FJ. Current recommendations for treatment of severe toxic alcohol poisonings. Intensive Care Med 2005;31:189–95.
31. Miott K, Striebel J, Cho AK, et al. Clinical and pharmacological aspects of bath salt use: a review of the literature and case reports. Drug Alcohol Depend 2013;132(1–2):1–12.
32. Terry SM. Bath salt abuse: more than just hot water. J Emerg Nurs 2014;40(1):88–91.
33. McGraw M, McGraw L. Bath salts: not as harmless as they sound. J Emerg Nurs 2012;38(6):582–8.
34. Salani DA, Zdanowicz MM. Synthetic cannabinoids: the dangers of spicing it up. J Psychosoc Nurs Ment Health Serv 2015;53(5):36–43.

35. Iman SF, Patel H, Mahmoud M, et al. Bath salts intoxication: a case series. J Emerg Med 2013;45(3):361–5.
36. Jordan JT, Harrison BE. Bath salts ingestion: diagnosis and treatment of substance-induced disorders. J Nurse Pract 2013;9(7):403–10.
37. Mills B, Yepes A, Nugent K. Synthetic cannabinoids. Am J Med Sci 2015;350(1): 59–62.
38. White CM. How MDMA's pharmacology and pharmacokinetics drive desired effects and harms. J Clin Pharmacol 2014;54(3):245–52.
39. Emde K. MDMA (ecstasy) in the emergency department. J Emerg Nurs 2003; 29(5):440–3.

Pharmacotherapy Considerations for the Management of Advanced Cardiac Life Support

Craig J. Beavers, PharmD, AACC, BCPS-AQ Cardiology*,
Komal A. Pandya, PharmD, BCPS

KEYWORDS

- Advanced cardiac life support • Vasopressin • Epinephrine • Cardiac arrest
- Ventricular fibrillation • Ventricular tachycardia

KEY POINTS

- It is critical that all members of the health care team have knowledge concerning the pharmacotherapy for advanced cardiac life support (ACLS).
- At present, vasopressin and epinephrine are the most commonly used agents in cardiac arrest.
- As resuscitation science evolves, potential changes to the treatment of ACLS could occur and providers should remain up to date on these changes.

INTRODUCTION

Sudden cardiac arrest (SCA) is defined as the failure of the heart to contract, and is evident by the loss of pulse.[1] The result is abrupt cessation of effective blood circulation leading to impaired oxygen delivery to vital organs. It is estimated that in 2014, 326,000 out-of-hospital cardiac arrests occurred, with a 10.6% survival rate.[2] An estimated 209,000 persons per year had in-hospital cardiac arrests, with a survival rate of 25.5%.[2] Given the time-sensitive nature of SCA, outcomes are improved when life-supporting measures occur rapidly on recognition.

Resuscitation science is ever evolving. The International Liaison Committee on Resuscitation (ILCOR), consisting of many stakeholders, including the American Heart

Disclosure: The authors and their spouses have no professional or financial disclosures, nor have they received any kind of support in the preparation of this article.
Department of Pharmacy Practice and Science, University of Kentucky UK Healthcare, Room H-110, 800 Rose Street, Lexington, KY 40536, USA
* Corresponding author.
E-mail address: cjbeav2@uky.edu

Nurs Clin N Am 51 (2016) 69–82
http://dx.doi.org/10.1016/j.cnur.2015.10.003
0029-6465/16/$ – see front matter © 2016 Elsevier Inc. All rights reserved.
nursing.theclinics.com

Association (AHA), focuses on fostering new research, evaluating new data, and publishing statements and guidelines regarding post-SCA resuscitation.[3] This organization develops and publishes new emergency cardiac care practice guidelines every 5 years. These recommendations become the basic life support (BLS) and advanced cardiac life support (ACLS) algorithms. The last updates were released in October 2015.[4]

These guidelines detail the critical elements in the management of patients with SCA to optimize chances of achieving return of spontaneous circulation (ROSC), survival to hospital admission, survival to discharge, overall survival, and survival with positive neurologic outcomes.[5] These components include cardiopulmonary resuscitation (CPR), including high-quality chest compressions, defibrillation, pharmacotherapy, therapeutic hypothermia, and postresuscitation management. This article highlights some key evidence regarding the pharmacotherapy for ventricular fibrillation (VF)/pulseless ventricular tachycardia (VT) and pulseless electrical activity (PEA)/asystole. The new adult cardiac support guidelines do not focus on bradyarrhythmias and tachyarrhythmias management strategies and thus are not discussed in this article. It is critical for all members of the health care team who care for patients with SCA to have an intimate knowledge regarding the pharmacologic agents that are used.

TYPES OF CARDIAC ARREST

SCA can be caused by any of 4 cardiac rhythms: VF, pulseless VT, PEA, or asystole. In general, VF is associated with disorganized electrical activity within the ventricular myocardium, whereas VT is more organized.[6] PEA represents a diverse group of organized rhythms that are associated with either lack of or insufficient ventricular activity in providing a perfusing rhythm or detectable pulse. Ventricular asystole refers to the absence of detectable ventricular electrical activity and pulse.[6] In this article, pulseless VT is referred to as VT.

Overall, management of these 4 rhythms is addressed with 2 treatment algorithms: 1 for VF/VT and 1 for PEA/asystole. No matter the type of rhythm involved, BLS (Fig. 1) and a coordinated, systematic method of providing ACLS are imperative to optimizing positive outcomes.[6,7] Although these management algorithms exist, it is important to understand that SCA can have many different causes and can occur in almost any type of situation (witnessed, unwitnessed, within the medical setting, or outside of the medical setting). Given this diversity, it is clear that a single approach to management is likely not ideal. However, a cohesive and consistent initial management strategy can help to guide subsequent management of the inciting factor. When these algorithms are implemented in a successful manner, survival rates after witnessed out-of hospital VF arrest approach 50% (range, 5%–50%).[6]

GOALS OF ADVANCED CARDIAC LIFE SUPPORT

The overarching goal of ACLS is for the patient to survive neurologically intact. In order to reach this goal, providers and possibly bystanders need to be rapid responders and proficient in the BLS and ACLS algorithms.[13] By following these guidelines, several short-term goals are highlighted: (1) early CPR and defibrillation; (2) achieving adequate coronary perfusion pressure (CPP), measured via arterial relaxation (diastolic) pressure; (3) achieving adequate cerebral blood flow; (4) ROSC; (5) survival to hospital admission; (6) stabilization of the patient; (7) appropriate post-code management; (8) prevention of future SCA events.[13]

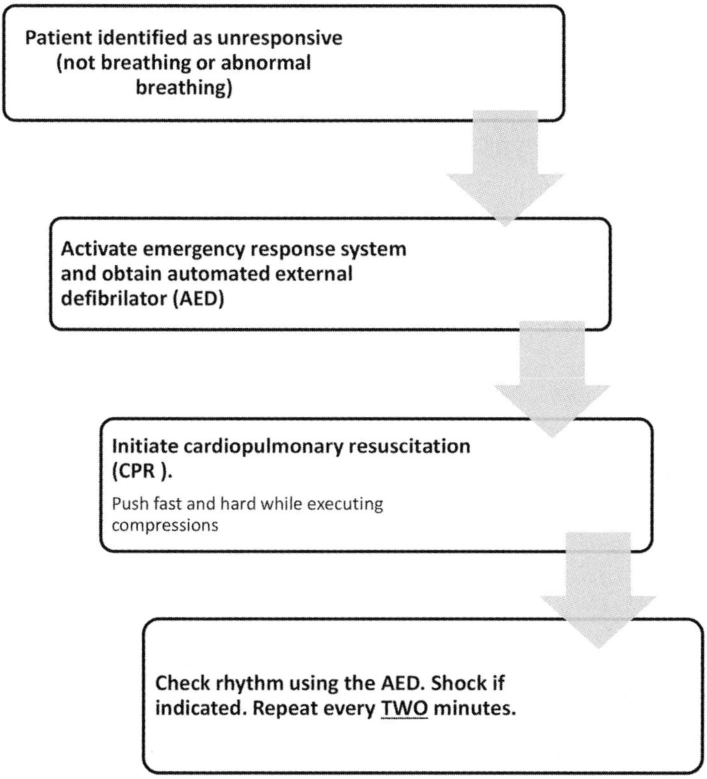

Fig. 1. BLS (adult). BLS represents the fundamental basis of SCA management. It stresses immediate recognition of SCA, activation of the emergency response system, initiation of CPR, and rapid defibrillation when appropriate. When done appropriately, chest compressions can increase intrathoracic pressure and apply force directly to the heart to circulate blood to vital organs. SCA responders should (1) push hard to a depth of 5 cm at a rate of 100 compressions per minute while ensuring that complete recoil of the chest occurs between compressions; (2) minimize interruptions in compressions; (3) target compression/ventilation ratio is 30:2 when giving rescue breathes. A prospective, population-based, observational study examined patients with SCA who underwent compression-only CPR and found that they had a higher rate of 1-year survival with favorable neurologic outcome compared with those that received no bystander CPR for out-of-hospital cardiac arrest (4.3% vs 2.5%; odds ratio, 1.72; 95% confidence interval, 1.01–2.95).[8] Conventional CPR showed similar effectiveness. Many other studies have validated these results.[9–12] The quality of CPR can be monitored with end-tidal CO_2 monitoring with a goal of greater than 10 mm Hg or diastolic arterial pressure greater than 20 mm Hg. Another important component of BLS is provision of defibrillation for shockable rhythms (VF/VT) because this provides a survival benefit. (*Data from* Kleinman ME, Brennan EE, Goldberger ZD, et al. Part 5: adult basic life support: 2015 American Heart Association guidelines for cardiopulmonary resuscitation and emergency cardiovascular care. Circulation 2015;132:S414–35.)

VENTRICULAR FIBRILLATION/VENTRICULAR TACHYCARDIA

The pharmacotherapy used during ACLS may not provide a long-term survival benefit without neurologic deficit, but does increase the chances of ROSC and survival to hospital admission. A variety of agents have been studied in the management of VF/VT (**Fig. 2**).[6]

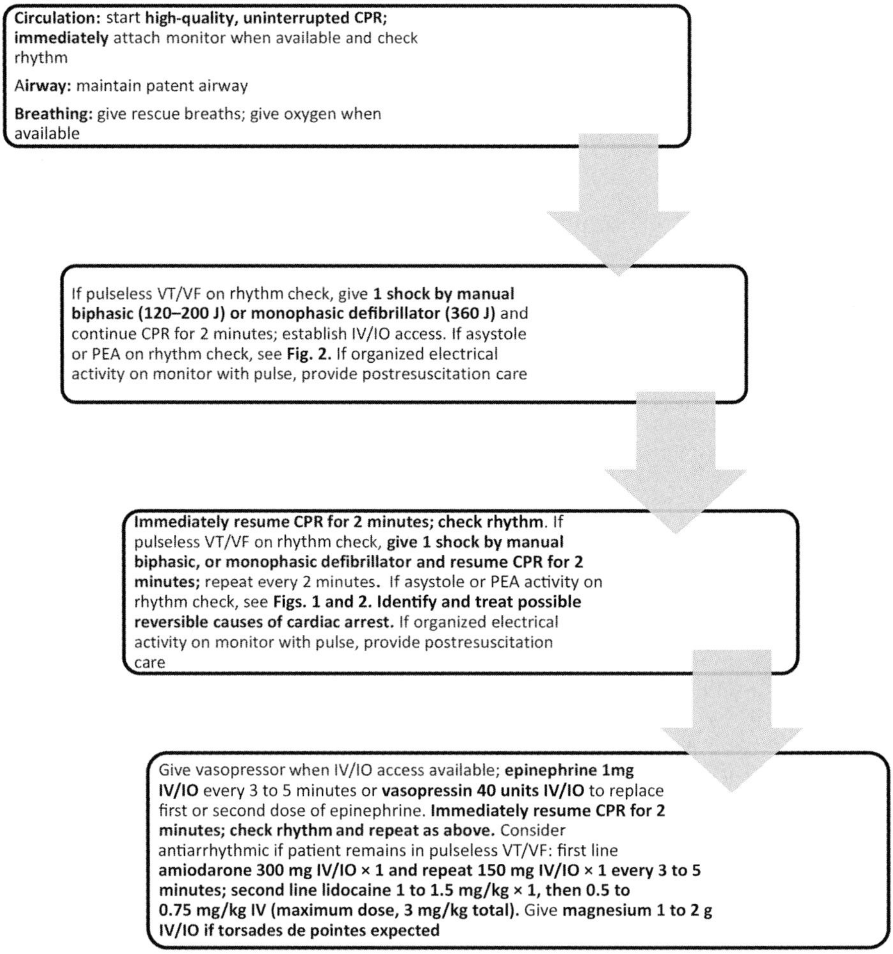

Circulation: start **high-quality, uninterrupted CPR; immediately** attach monitor when available and check rhythm

Airway: maintain patent airway

Breathing: give rescue breaths; give oxygen when available

If pulseless VT/VF on rhythm check, give **1 shock by manual biphasic (120–200 J) or monophasic defibrillator (360 J)** and continue CPR for 2 minutes; establish IV/IO access. If asystole or PEA on rhythm check, see **Fig. 2.** If organized electrical activity on monitor with pulse, provide postresuscitation care

Immediately resume CPR for 2 minutes; check rhythm. If pulseless VT/VF on rhythm check, **give 1 shock by manual biphasic, or monophasic defibrillator and resume CPR for 2 minutes;** repeat every 2 minutes. If asystole or PEA activity on rhythm check, see **Figs. 1 and 2. Identify and treat possible reversible causes of cardiac arrest.** If organized electrical activity on monitor with pulse, provide postresuscitation care

Give vasopressor when IV/IO access available; **epinephrine 1mg IV/IO** every 3 to 5 minutes or **vasopressin 40 units IV/IO** to replace first or second dose of epinephrine. **Immediately resume CPR for 2 minutes; check rhythm and repeat as above.** Consider antiarrhythmic if patient remains in pulseless VT/VF: first line **amiodarone 300 mg IV/IO × 1 and repeat 150 mg IV/IO × 1 every 3 to 5 minutes; second line lidocaine 1 to 1.5 mg/kg × 1, then 0.5 to 0.75 mg/kg IV (maximum dose, 3 mg/kg total).** Give magnesium 1 to 2 g IV/IO if torsades de pointes expected

Fig. 2. VF/pulseless VT algorithm. IO, intraosseous; IV, intravenous. (*Data from* Link MS, Berkow LC, Kudenchuk PJ, et al. Part 7: adult advanced cardiovascular life support: 2015 American Heart Association guidelines for cardiopulmonary resuscitation and emergency cardiovascular care. Circulation 2015;132:S444–64.)

Based on available clinical evidence, the 2015 AHA ACLS guidelines recommend administration of epinephrine solely when VF/VT persists after 1 defibrillation attempt and a round of 2 minutes of CPR and removal of the use of vasopressin.[6] Vasopressors are thought to promote adequate CPP, defined by the pressure gradient between diastolic aortic pressure and left ventricular end-diastolic pressure. The resulting CPP support results in optimization of coronary blood flow, leading to successful oxygenation, defibrillation, and ultimately ROSC.[13]

The discovery that the human body releases endogenously synthesized vasoconstricting substances that affect CPP set the foundation to further explore the utility of vasopressors in this setting. Most research regarding vasopressor use in cardiac arrest focuses on the use of epinephrine, vasopressin, or the combination of both. However, despite guideline recommendations and frequent use, there is still clinical uncertainty about the optimal agent, dose, timing, administration sequence, and number of doses for the best outcomes.

Epinephrine

Epinephrine is a naturally occurring vasoconstricting compound that stimulates the α-adrenergic receptor on vascular smooth muscle, leading to arterial vasoconstriction, improved coronary blood flow, and CPP.[14] Although these effects are positive, epinephrine also targets β-adrenergic receptors on myocardial tissue, which can cause a dose-dependent increase in myocardial oxygen demand that is likely to be greater than what is supplied, resulting in lactic acid development.[15]

Administration of epinephrine increases rates of ROSC from 30% to 38%. However, it does not improve survival to hospital discharge.[6] Potential limitations to the evidence include the lack of adequate randomized controlled trials comparing it with placebo. Limited data suggest that epinephrine may be harmful if administration is given later during resuscitation efforts.[16] Furthermore, there has been much debate regarding the optimal dose.

Because of the worsening acidosis that occurs with diminished perfusion, the risk of a blunted response of adrenergic agents theoretically occurs.[14,15] Because of this phenomenon, several studies have examined the use of high doses (up to 10 mg or 0.2 mg/kg), compared with lower, standard doses (1 mg).[17–20] Several studies compared high-dose epinephrine with standard dose and found no difference in ROSC, immediate survival, overall successful resuscitation, or survival to hospital discharge.[17,18,20] A meta-analysis showed that high-dose epinephrine improved ROSC with no difference in survival outcomes.[19] The largest trial examining higher doses explored patients with VF, PEA, or asystole and randomized them to 5 mg versus 1 mg (with 15 mg maximum cumulative dose).[21] Overall, the rate of ROSC (40.6% vs 36.4%; $P = .02$) and survival to hospital admission (26.5% vs 23.5%; $P = .05$) were improved in the high-dose group with no difference in survival with favorable neurologic outcome and survival to discharge.[21] On review of subgroups, the investigators noted that patients who had VF as their initial rhythm were less likely to achieve ROSC and survival to hospital admission.[21] Investigators observed no benefit derived from higher doses in patients with defibrillation-refractory rhythms.[21]

Given the lack of benefit on long-term survival, the potential for demand ischemia, and possible postresuscitation adverse effects (eg, tachycardia, hypertension, myocardial dysfunction), the 2015 AHA guidelines state that it is reasonable to use the 1-mg dose via the intravenous (IV)/intraosseous (IO) route every 3 to 5 minutes during cardiac arrest.[6] However, they recommend consideration for higher doses in situations such as β-blocker/calcium channel blocker overdose, endotracheal administration, or if hemodynamic monitoring of arterial relaxation pressure or CPP occurs.[6]

Given the many questions remaining with regard to epinephrine, there is a clear need to have focused efforts to research its role, administration timing, and dosing.

Vasopressin

Vasopressin is a nonadrenergic neuropeptide hormone that causes peripheral, coronary, and renal artery vasoconstriction via interaction with V1 receptor on smooth muscle cells.[15] Compared with epinephrine, vasopressin has a gradual onset and longer half-life.[14] Evidence from 3 randomized controlled trials and 1 meta-analysis shows no difference in the outcomes of ROSC, survival to discharge, or survival with favorable neurologic outcomes between IV vasopressin 40 units or epinephrine 1 mg as a first-line vasopressor (**Table 1**).[22–25]

Table 1
Prospective, multicenter, double-blind, randomized controlled trials of vasopressin in cardiac arrest

Authors	Study Population (n)	Setting	Intervention in Vasopressin Group, Dose of Vasopressin[a]	Intervention in Control Group[a]	Initial Cardiac Rhythm (%)	Primary End Points Vasopressin Versus Control
Stiell et al,[24] 2001	Adult patients (≥16 y old) with cardiac arrest (n = 200)	In hospital	Vasopressin followed by EPI, 40 IU	EPI and placebo	VF/VT: 21 PEA: 48 Asystole: 31	Survival to hospital discharge: 12% vs 14%, P = .67 Survival to 1 h: 39% vs 35%, P = .66 Neurologic function by MMES score: 36 vs 35, P = .75
Wenzel et al,[25] 2004	Adult patients (≥18 y old) with cardiac arrest (n = 1186)	Out of hospital	Vasopressin followed by EPI, 40–80 IU	EPI and placebo	VT/VF: 40 PEA: 16 Asystole: 45	Survival to hospital admission: 46.2% vs 43.0%, P = .48
Callaway et al,[23] 2006	Adult patients (≥18 y old) with cardiac arrest (n = 325)	Out of hospital	Vasopressin and EPI, 40–80 IU	EPI and placebo	VF/VT: 15 PEA: 22 Asystole: 51	ROSC at any time during resuscitation: 31% vs 30%, P = .88 Presence of pulses at hospital arrival: 19% vs 23%, P = .28
Gueugniaud et al,[26] 2008	Adult patients (≥18 y old) with cardiac arrest (n = 2984)	Out of hospital	Vasopressin and EPI, 40–80 IU	EPI and placebo	VF/VT: 9 PEA: 8 Asystole: 83	Survival to hospital admission: 20.7% vs 21.3%, P = .69

Abbreviations: EPI, epinephrine; IU, international units; MMES, mini-mental status examination score; PEA, pulseless electrical activity; ROSC, return of spontaneous circulation; VASO, vasopressin; VF, ventricular fibrillation; vs, versus; VT, ventricular tachycardia.
[a] drugs were administered exclusively intravenously in all studies.

A trial exploring the impact of repeated administration of vasopressin and epinephrine in patients with out-of-hospital arrest receiving prolonged CPR was conducted.[26] Each group received up to 4 injections of either 40 units of vasopressin (n = 137) or 1 mg of epinephrine (n = 118). Investigators found no difference in ROSC (28.7% vs 26.6%; P = .743), 24-hour survival (16.9% vs 20.3%; P = .468), and survival to hospital discharge (5.8% vs 4.2%; P = .560).[26] Mukoyama and colleagues[27] released a study in 2009 that explored the effectiveness of repeated doses of vasopressin versus epinephrine. The primary outcome was survival to hospital discharge with good neurologic outcome. Secondary outcomes included ROSC and 24-hour survival. Overall, there were no statistically significant differences between any of the outcomes examined, suggesting that epinephrine is equivalent to vasopressin.

Given the collective quality of data, the 2015 AHA guidelines recommend against the administration of 40 units of vasopressin as a single-dose alternative to epinephrine during the first or second round of medication administration during ACLS, which is a drastic change from previous guidelines.[6]

Steroids with Vasopressors

Recent interest has developed in exploring the use of steroids in combination with vasopressors. Mentzelopoulos and colleagues[28] recently published a randomized, double-blind, placebo-controlled, parallel-group trial, the largest to date, to determine whether a combination of vasopressin, epinephrine, and methylprednisolone 40 mg supplementation during in-hospital cardiac arrest improved survival to hospital discharge with favorable neurologic outcome. Postresuscitation, these patients received hydrocortisone 300 mg intravenously daily for less than or equal to 7 days followed by a gradual taper. Patients receiving the combination of medications had a higher probability of achieving ROSC for 20 minutes or longer (109 of 130 [83.9%] vs 91 of 138 [65.9%]; odds ratio [OR], 2.98; 95% confidence interval [CI], 1.39–6.40; P = .005). Furthermore, those receiving the combination were more likely to survive to hospital discharge with favorable neurologic outcome (18 of 130 [13.9%] vs 7 of 138 [5.1%]; OR, 3.28; 95% CI, 1.17–9.20; P = .02). Despite these data, the 2015 guidelines did not consider that the evidence was strong enough for support for or against the routine use of steroids in conjunction with vasopressors; however, they do acknowledge that they may be considered.[6] If this strategy is used, it is recommend the dosing and selection of agents be similar to those used in the Mentzelopoulos and colleagues[28] trial.

Antiarrhythmics

Antiarrhythmics have not been shown to improve long-term survival. However, they are administered to prevent further episodes of VT/VF and improve ROSC. The 2015 AHA guidelines recommend the use of a single antiarrhythmic in patients with VF/VT to eliminate the potential for adverse events.[6] At present, recommended agents are amiodarone and lidocaine. Magnesium sulfate is also recommended but use is limited to torsades de pointes associated with a prolonged QT interval.[6]

Amiodarone

Amiodarone possesses potassium channel, calcium channel, sodium channel, and α-blocking and β-blocking properties.[15] Originally indicated for management of recurrent VT, 2 large, randomized controlled trials have caused it to be accepted into ACLS management with demonstrated improvements in ROSC and survival to hospital admission.[29,30] In the Amiodarone for Resuscitation After Out-of-Hospital Cardiac Arrest due to VF (ARREST) trial, 504 patients with out-of-hospital cardiac arrest, VT/VF, who were not resuscitated after 3 automated external defibrillator shocks, and who received 1 mg of epinephrine, were randomized to IV amiodarone 300 mg (n = 246) or placebo (n = 258).[30] Significantly more patients in the amiodarone group survived to hospital admission with ROSC (44% vs 33%; P = .03). However, there was no difference in survival to hospital discharge.[30] More patients in the amiodarone group had hypotension and bradycardia caused by the solvents in the formation (polysorbate 80 and benzyl alcohol).[29] In the Amiodarone versus Lidocaine in Pre-hospital VF Evaluation (ALIVE) trial, amiodarone was compared with lidocaine in 347 patients who had VF resistant to 3 shocks, IV epinephrine, and a further shock or VF that reoccurred after successful defibrillation.[29] Investigators observed a higher rate of survival to hospital admission with amiodarone compared with lidocaine (22.8% vs 12.0%; P = .009) if the drug was administered in the first 24 minutes only.[29]

The 2015 AHA guidelines recommend administration of 300 mg of amiodarone followed by a supplemental 150-mg dose if the patient is not successfully resuscitated via CPR, defibrillation, and epinephrine.[6] The 2015 guidelines found insufficient evidence for or against routine initiation or continuation of amiodarone after ROSC after cardiac arrest and this is left up to the health care team.[6]

Lidocaine

Historically, lidocaine was the antiarrhythmic of choice for the management of SCA because of the perception of lower rates of adverse effects compared with alternative agents.[6] However, the evidence proving any form of benefit has not been validated in the literature. Because amiodarone has been found to be superior in the literature, lidocaine became the second-line agent for the management of refractory VF/VT in the 2015 AHA guidelines and should only be used if amiodarone is unavailable.[6] If lidocaine is used, the initial dose should be 1 to 1.5 mg/kg and repeat doses of 0.5 to 0.75 mg/kg every 5 to 10 minutes to a total loading dose of up to 3 mg/kg. The 2015 guidelines could find evidence for continuation of lidocaine, if used in place of amiodarone, after ROSC.[15] Typically, lidocaine is administered via continuous infusion at 1 to 4 mg/min. Lower rates of infusion should be used in patients with hepatic or renal failure to limit or avoid neurologic side effects.[15]

Magnesium Sulfate

The administration of magnesium sulfate has proved to be effective at terminating torsades de pointes, a variant of polymorphic VT with a prolonged QT interval, in 2 observational studies.[6,31] However, use of magnesium for other forms of VF/VT with a normal QT interval has not been shown to affect outcomes.[32–34] The 2015 AHA guidelines suggest that magnesium should be given as an IV bolus of 1 to 2 g only during clear cases of torsades.[6] The optimal dosing or maximal threshold dosing in torsades has not been established via clinical trials and is mostly related to antidotal experience.[6]

THERAPIES NO LONGER RECOMMENDED DURING CARDIAC ARREST

As resuscitation science evolves, many agents once commonly used during SCA cease to be the standard of care. Agents such as sodium bicarbonate, atropine, and calcium chloride are, outside of specific situations, no longer routinely recommended.[6]

Sodium Bicarbonate

Historically, sodium bicarbonate was given to treat the acidosis that is commonly caused by hypoperfusion during SCA. Theoretically, it reverses negative effects on impaired receptor responsiveness in conditions of acidosis and myocardial contractility that occur in an acidotic environment.[13] However, data from 2 prospective randomized controlled trials have shown no benefit.[35,36] In the first trial, 502 out-of-hospital patients with VF and asystolic arrest were given a buffered solution containing either sodium bicarbonate or 0.9% sodium chloride.[33] The investigators found no difference in ROSC or survival to discharge.[35] In the second trial, 874 patients with out-of-hospital arrest were given 1 mEq/kg of sodium bicarbonate or placebo after several rounds of CPR.[36] There was no difference in survival between the two groups. Therefore, the 2015 guidelines strongly discourage the use of sodium bicarbonate routinely in ACLS unless there is a clear indication such as hyperkalemia, preexisting sodium bicarbonate-responsive acidosis, tricyclic depression overdose, intubation and mechanical ventilation with prolonged arrest interval, or in patients who have ROSC after prolonged arrest.[6]

Atropine

Despite being included in previous iterations of the PEA/asystole algorithm, atropine has been removed from the most recent guidelines.[6] The impetus for the change was the lack of high-quality, prospective controlled trials examining atropine in bradycardic PEA/asystole.[6] The recommendation from past guidelines came from low-quality trials that provided conflicting evidence. Overall, there lacks current evidence to suggest that atropine is likely to have a benefit and it should not be used in cardiac arrest.[6]

Calcium Chloride

Routine administration of calcium during ACLS has been deemed of no benefit in the 2015 guidelines and is not recommend (III/B).[6] The evidence for calcium has been variable in terms of ROSC for survival during in-hospital or out-hospital arrest. The guidelines do recommend calcium to be administered during situations of hyperkalemia with electrocardiogram changes using 10% calcium chloride 500 to 1000 mg (5–10 mL) IV over 2 to 5 minutes in conjunction with dextrose and insulin.[6] If the patient lacks central line access, calcium gluconate is preferred to limit phlebitis.[14]

PULSELESS ELECTRICAL ACTIVITY AND ASYSTOLE

Similar to VF/VT management, to date no placebo-controlled trial has shown that administration of any vasopressor results in increased chances of neurologically intact survival. Instead, use of vasopressors is associated with an increased rate of achieving ROSC, which allows health care teams to determine the cause of SCA and implement measures to address those causes. Also similar to VF/VT, adequate CPR is a key initial management strategy (**Fig. 3**).[6]

The mainstay of pharmacologic therapy in patients with PEA/asystole is epinephrine.[6] One study by Jacobs and colleagues[37] in 2011 compared 1 mg epinephrine every 3 minutes with placebo in 534 subjects in a double-blind, randomized, placebo-controlled trial. Outcomes examined included achievement of ROSC, survival to hospital discharge (which was the primary end point), and a neurologic outcome. For patients administered epinephrine, the likelihood of achieving ROSC prehospital was 3.4 times greater than for those receiving placebo. Epinephrine was also associated with a significant increase in the proportion of patients admitted to hospital. Good neurologic outcome was achieved in 14 of 16 survivors.[35] The treatment effect of epinephrine on prehospital ROSC was more marked in nonshockable rhythms (PEA/asystole) than shockable rhythms.

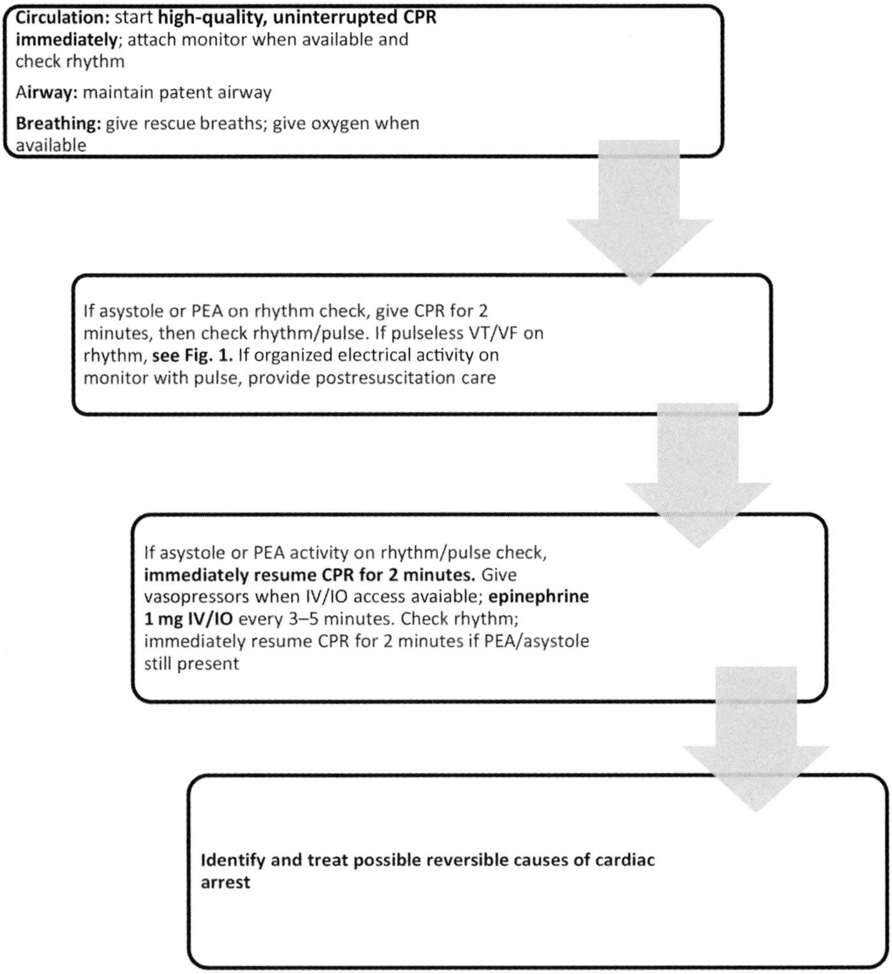

Circulation: start **high-quality, uninterrupted CPR immediately**; attach monitor when available and check rhythm

Airway: maintain patent airway

Breathing: give rescue breaths; give oxygen when available

If asystole or PEA on rhythm check, give CPR for 2 minutes, then check rhythm/pulse. If pulseless VT/VF on rhythm, **see Fig. 1.** If organized electrical activity on monitor with pulse, provide postresuscitation care

If asystole or PEA activity on rhythm/pulse check, **immediately resume CPR for 2 minutes.** Give vasopressors when IV/IO access avaiable; **epinephrine 1 mg IV/IO** every 3–5 minutes. Check rhythm; immediately resume CPR for 2 minutes if PEA/asystole still present

Identify and treat possible reversible causes of cardiac arrest

Fig. 3. PEA/asystole algorithm. (*Data from* Link MS, Berkow LC, Kudenchuk PJ, et al. Part 7: adult advanced cardiovascular life support: 2015 American Heart Association guidelines for cardiopulmonary resuscitation and emergency cardiovascular care. Circulation 2015;132:S444–64.)

It is common for patients to present with one rhythm and, during the course of resuscitation, show a different rhythm. For example, a patient may initially present with VT/VF, be defibrillated, and then convert to PEA/asystole. Providers should always be on the lookout for changes in rhythms and shift their management strategy appropriately.

POST-CODE MANAGEMENT

The importance of post-code care for patients who experience ROSC and survive cardiac arrest is becoming more apparent.[38,39] Following a cardiac arrest, the myocardium begins to recover from ischemia and acidosis. Patients are at increased risk of developing the various types of shock, systemic inflammatory response syndrome, and sepsis, and are likely to have had perfusion-related injury

Table 2	
Possible reversible causes for cardiac arrest	
Hs	**Ts**
Hypoxia	Toxins
Hypovolemia	Tamponade (cardiac)
Hydrogen ions (acidosis)	Tension pneumothorax
Hypokalemia/hyperkalemia	Thrombosis (pulmonary embolism)
Hypothermia	Thrombosis (coronary)

to vital organs.[38] The objectives of post-code management are to (1) optimize cardiopulmonary function and vital organ perfusion, (2) relocate the patient to a setting that allows for comprehensive care of the underlying SCA cause, (3) identification and treatment of the causes of the SCA event to prevent further events, and (4) control body temperature to promote neurologic recovery.[39] Readers are encouraged to review the section of the 2010 guidelines regarding post-code management for more detail.[39]

Vasopressor and antiarrhythmic agents are administered in post-code settings to provide hemodynamic support, assist with cardiac output, and prevent recurrent events with the aim of avoiding hypotension (systolic blood pressure <90 mm Hg, mean arterial pressure <65 mm Hg).[38] There is no specific agent to recommend as first line in this setting. The choice of agent is driven anecdotally by hemodynamic response and adverse events.[13] An ideal suggested range of doses for these medications cannot be established because of the change in pharmacokinetics of these agents in settings of poor perfusion, organ injury, potential for hypothermia, and acidosis.[14,38,40] In general, therapy is titrated based on patient response and hemodynamic demands. Note that vasoactive agents, such as epinephrine and norepinephrine, should be administered via a central line whenever possible because of the risk of tissue necrosis if extravasation occurs.[13] In addition, in the setting of therapeutic hypothermia, the pharmacokinetics and pharmacodynamics of many drugs can be significantly altered, possibly resulting in alterations in response to these agents and the potential to result in adverse events.[41] Consultation with a clinical pharmacist to assist in the proper dosing and management of pharmacotherapy in patients undergoing therapeutic hypothermia is recommended.

Both during and after the management of SCA, health care providers should consider the Hs and Ts to identify and manage any common risk factors that may have contributed to the arrest (**Table 2**).[42] Additional pharmacologic therapies may be used if any of these risk factors (eg, thrombus) are identified.

SUMMARY

When a patient has a cardiac arrest, it is critical that providers have mastery of the cardiac arrest algorithms and understand the pharmacotherapy used. Although medication therapy has not been proved to reduce mortality, understanding the rationale and dosing of therapy can prevent unnecessary harm. It is imperative that clinicians provide proper treatment in the postresuscitation period to prevent future events. In addition, as research provides new insight into the management of cardiac arrest, health care professionals should keep abreast of the evidence and guideline changes.

REFERENCES

1. Kasper DL, Harrison TR. Harrison's principles of internal medicine. 16th edition. New York: McGraw-Hill, Medical Pub Division; 2005.
2. Mozaffarian D, Benjamin EJ, Go AS, et al. Heart disease and stroke statistics–2015 update: a report from the American Heart Association. Circulation 2015; 131:e29–322.
3. Morrison LJ, Gent LM, Lang E, et al. Part 2: evidence evaluation and management of conflicts of interest: 2015 American Heart Association guidelines for cardiopulmonary resuscitation and emergency cardiovascular care. Circulation 2015;132:S368–82.
4. ILCOR-Home. 2015. Available at: http://www.ilcor.org/home/. Accessed June 20th, 2015 and October 15, 2015.
5. Neumar RW, Shuster M, Callaway CW, et al. Part 1: executive summary: 2015 American Heart Association guidelines for cardiopulmonary resuscitation and emergency cardiovascular care. Circulation 2015;132:S315–67.
6. Link MS, Berkow LC, Kudenchuk PJ, et al. Part 7: adult advanced cardiovascular life support: 2015 American Heart Association guidelines for cardiopulmonary resuscitation and emergency cardiovascular care. Circulation 2015;132:S444–64.
7. Kleinman ME, Brennan EE, Goldberger ZD, et al. Part 5: adult basic life support: 2015 American Heart Association guidelines for cardiopulmonary resuscitation and emergency cardiovascular care. Circulation 2015;132:S414–35.
8. Iwami T, Kawamura T, Hiraide A, et al. Effectiveness of bystander-initiated cardiac-only resuscitation for patients with out-of-hospital cardiac arrest. Circulation 2007;116:2900–7.
9. Bohm K, Rosenqvist M, Herlitz J, et al. Survival is similar after standard treatment and chest compression only in out-of-hospital bystander cardiopulmonary resuscitation. Circulation 2007;116:2908–12.
10. SOS-KANTO Study Group. Cardiopulmonary resuscitation by bystanders with chest compression only (SOS-KANTO): an observational study. Lancet 2007; 369:920–6.
11. Olasveengen TM, Wik L, Steen PA. Standard basic life support vs. continuous chest compressions only in out-of-hospital cardiac arrest. Acta Anaesthesiol Scand 2008;52:914–9.
12. Ong ME, Ng FS, Anushia P, et al. Comparison of chest compression only and standard cardiopulmonary resuscitation for out-of-hospital cardiac arrest in Singapore. Resuscitation 2008;78:119–26.
13. Hesch K. Cardiac arrest and advanced cardiac life support in pharmacotherapy self-assessment program: critical and urgent care. In: Lenexa KS, editor. PSAP 2014 edition. Lenexa (KS): American College of Clinical Pharmacy; 2014. p. 3–30.
14. Wiggins BS, Sanoski CA, American Society of Health-System Pharmacists. Emergency cardiovascular pharmacotherapy: a point-of-care guide. Bethesda (MD): American Society of Health-System Pharmacists; 2012.
15. Dager WE, Sanoski CA, Wiggins BS, et al. Pharmacotherapy considerations in advanced cardiac life support. Pharmacotherapy 2006;26:1703–29.
16. Dumas F, Bougouin W, Geri G, et al. Is epinephrine during cardiac arrest associated with worse outcomes in resuscitated patients? J Am Coll Cardiol 2014;64: 2360–7.
17. Brown CG, Martin DR, Pepe PE, et al. A comparison of standard-dose and high-dose epinephrine in cardiac arrest outside the hospital. The Multicenter High-Dose Epinephrine Study Group. N Engl J Med 1992;327:1051–5.

18. Stiell IG, Hebert PC, Weitzman BN, et al. High-dose epinephrine in adult cardiac arrest. N Engl J Med 1992;327:1045–50.
19. Vandycke C, Martens P. High dose versus standard dose epinephrine in cardiac arrest - a meta-analysis. Resuscitation 2000;45:161–6.
20. Woodhouse SP, Cox S, Boyd P, et al. High dose and standard dose adrenaline do not alter survival, compared with placebo, in cardiac arrest. Resuscitation 1995; 30:243–9.
21. Gueugniaud PY, Mols P, Goldstein P, et al. A comparison of repeated high doses and repeated standard doses of epinephrine for cardiac arrest outside the hospital. European Epinephrine Study Group. N Engl J Med 1998;339:1595–601.
22. Aung K, Htay T. Vasopressin for cardiac arrest: a systematic review and meta-analysis. Arch Intern Med 2005;165:17–24.
23. Callaway CW, Hostler D, Doshi AA, et al. Usefulness of vasopressin administered with epinephrine during out-of-hospital cardiac arrest. Am J Cardiol 2006;98: 1316–21.
24. Stiell IG, Hebert PC, Wells GA, et al. Vasopressin versus epinephrine for inhospital cardiac arrest: a randomised controlled trial. Lancet 2001;358:105–9.
25. Wenzel V, Krismer AC, Arntz HR, et al. A comparison of vasopressin and epinephrine for out-of-hospital cardiopulmonary resuscitation. N Engl J Med 2004;350: 105–13.
26. Gueugniaud PY, David JS, Chanzy E, et al. Vasopressin and epinephrine vs. epinephrine alone in cardiopulmonary resuscitation. N Engl J Med 2008;359: 21–30.
27. Mukoyama T, Kinoshita K, Nagao K, et al. Reduced effectiveness of vasopressin in repeated doses for patients undergoing prolonged cardiopulmonary resuscitation. Resuscitation 2009;80:755–61.
28. Mentzelopoulos SD, Malachias S, Chamos C, et al. Vasopressin, steroids, and epinephrine and neurologically favorable survival after in-hospital cardiac arrest: a randomized clinical trial. JAMA 2013;310:270–9.
29. Dorian P, Cass D, Schwartz B, et al. Amiodarone as compared with lidocaine for shock-resistant ventricular fibrillation. N Engl J Med 2002;346:884–90.
30. Kudenchuk PJ, Cobb LA, Copass MK, et al. Amiodarone for resuscitation after out-of-hospital cardiac arrest due to ventricular fibrillation. N Engl J Med 1999; 341:871–8.
31. Tzivoni D, Banai S, Schuger C, et al. Treatment of torsade de pointes with magnesium sulfate. Circulation 1988;77:392–7.
32. Allegra J, Lavery R, Cody R, et al. Magnesium sulfate in the treatment of refractory ventricular fibrillation in the prehospital setting. Resuscitation 2001;49:245–9.
33. Fatovich DM, Prentice DA, Dobb GJ. Magnesium in cardiac arrest (the magic trial). Resuscitation 1997;35:237–41.
34. Thel MC, Armstrong AL, McNulty SE, et al. Randomised trial of magnesium in in-hospital cardiac arrest. Duke Internal Medicine Housestaff. Lancet 1997;350: 1272–6.
35. Dybvik T, Strand T, Steen PA. Buffer therapy during out-of-hospital cardiopulmonary resuscitation. Resuscitation 1995;29:89–95.
36. Vukmir RB, Katz L, Sodium Bicarbonate Study Group. Sodium bicarbonate improves outcome in prolonged prehospital cardiac arrest. Am J Emerg Med 2006;24:156–61.
37. Jacobs IG, Finn JC, Jelinek GA, et al. Effect of adrenaline on survival in out-of-hospital cardiac arrest: A randomised double-blind placebo-controlled trial. Resuscitation 2011;82:1138–43.

38. Neumar RW, Nolan JP, Adrie C, et al. Post-cardiac arrest syndrome: epidemiology, pathophysiology, treatment, and prognostication. A consensus statement from the International Liaison Committee on Resuscitation (American Heart Association, Australian and New Zealand Council on Resuscitation, European Resuscitation Council, Heart and Stroke Foundation of Canada, InterAmerican Heart Foundation, Resuscitation Council of Asia, and the Resuscitation Council of Southern Africa); the American Heart Association Emergency Cardiovascular Care Committee; the Council on Cardiovascular Surgery and Anesthesia; the Council on Cardiopulmonary, Perioperative, and Critical Care; the Council on Clinical Cardiology; and the Stroke Council. Circulation 2008;118:2452–83.
39. Callaway CW, Donnino MW, Fink EL, et al. Part 8: post-cardiac arrest care: 2015 American Heart Association guidelines for cardiopulmonary resuscitation and emergency cardiovascular care. Circulation 2015;132:S465–82.
40. Kellum JA, Pinsky MR. Use of vasopressor agents in critically ill patients. Curr Opin Crit Care 2002;8:236–41.
41. Arpino PA, Greer DM. Practical pharmacologic aspects of therapeutic hypothermia after cardiac arrest. Pharmacotherapy 2008;28:102–11.
42. Lavonas EJ, Drennan IR, Gabrielli A, et al. Part 10: cardiac arrest in special situations: 2015 American Heart Association guidelines for cardiopulmonary resuscitation and emergency cardiovascular care. Circulation 2015;132: S501–18.

Blood Transfusion Strategies for Hemostatic Resuscitation in Massive Trauma

CrossMark

Caroline McGrath, DNP, CRNA*

KEYWORDS

- Lethal triad • Trauma • Hemorrhage • Whole blood • 1:1:1 component therapy
- Hemostatic resuscitation • Massive transfusion protocol

KEY POINTS

- Nonhemostatic resuscitation in the face of preventable massive hemorrhage results in a greater than 40% mortality rate.
- Forty years ago blood transfusion practice moved from fresh whole blood to stored components without evidence comparing the benefits or risks of either approach.
- Fresh whole blood has demonstrated superior effectiveness in treating early or acute coagulopathy of trauma in studies from the most recent theaters of war.
- The blood transfusion practices modified by the US military have guided recent massive transfusion protocols (MTP) in civilian trauma facilities.
- Prospective, randomized trials are needed in civilian trauma centers to determine whether one resuscitation strategy is superior to the other.

INTRODUCTION

Hemorrhage is the major preventable cause of mortality among trauma patients with otherwise survivable injuries.[1] Trauma involving blood loss of greater than 40% blood volume is often associated with irreversible hemorrhagic shock. Collectively referred to as "the lethal triad," irreversible physiologic derangements of acidosis, hypothermia, and coagulopathy lead to death in more than 50% of patients with hemorrhagic shock despite appropriate trauma care and multiple blood transfusions.[1,2]

Forty years ago, blood transfusion was largely dependent on the use of whole blood. In the 1970s, transfusion procedures within civilian trauma practices switched from the use of whole blood to predominantly conventional component therapy following development of whole blood fractionation.[3–5] Conventional component therapy is

Disclosure: None.
School of Nursing, Vanderbilt University, Nashville, TN, USA
* 1726 Bolton Village Lane, Niceville, FL 32578.
E-mail addresses: caroline.mcgrath@vanderbilt.edu; caroline.mcgrath.ccc@gmail.com

Nurs Clin N Am 51 (2016) 83–93
http://dx.doi.org/10.1016/j.cnur.2015.11.001
0029-6465/16/$ – see front matter Published by Elsevier Inc.

achieved by collecting whole blood from donors and processing the blood into separate red blood cells (RBC), platelets, and plasma components during fractionation. The change from whole blood to component transfusion occurred without evidence comparing the benefits or risks of either transfusion therapy among patients with traumatic hemorrhage.[6] After component therapy was instituted, transfusion goals consisted of normalizing blood pressure after trauma by infusing large volumes of crystalloid resuscitation. Standard therapy for any patient with suspected bleeding was a 2-L crystalloid bolus as initial therapy. Additional crystalloid boluses were often repeated and blood transfusion therapy was used relatively late in resuscitation. Fresh frozen plasma (FFP) and platelets were also used relatively late, often after patients had received 10 U of red cells. In this conventional component resuscitation, dilutional anemia persisted and patients with large-volume blood loss often died of what has been called a "bloody vicious cycle."[7]

The lethal triad, or bloody vicious cycle, is extremely difficult to reverse and is frequently worsened by nonhemostatic transfusion associated with conventional component therapy resuscitation.[8] Effective treatment of life-threatening hemorrhage, which corrects lethal triad derangements, could potentially eradicate death by exsanguination related to severe trauma. The military experiences in Iraq and Afghanistan forced the use of fresh whole blood (FWB) transfusion during shortages of component therapy and as a last ditch effort to reverse exsanguination. The overwhelming success with FWB in the war zone has prompted civilian trauma teams to advocate for this new technique of hemostatic resuscitation as a means to stop exsanguination for life-threatening hemorrhage.[4,8,9]

LETHAL TRIAD OF TRAUMA

The concept of the lethal triad (also known as the "trauma triad of death") is a medical term describing the combination of three subconcepts or components of the triad: acidosis, hypothermia, and coagulopathy (**Fig. 1**). Cumulative effects of each subconcept are commonly seen in patients who have sustained severe traumatic injuries and result in a significant rise in mortality rate. When a traumatized patient presents with the lethal triad, damage control surgery is required to reverse the effects. Damage control surgery involves only those procedures that provide rapid control of life-threatening bleeding followed by correction of physiologic abnormalities, associated

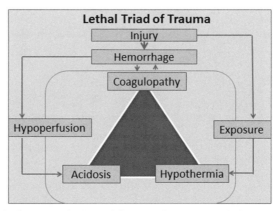

Fig. 1. Lethal triad of trauma. (*Adapted from* Dadhwal US, Pathak N. Damage control philosophy in polytrauma. Med J Armed Forces India 2010;66(4):348; with permission.)

with the lethal triad of hypothermia, acidosis, and coagulopathy before definitive management of injuries.[10]

These three conditions share a complex relationship with each factor compounding the others, resulting in high mortality if the cycle continues uninterrupted.[11] Interruption of the lethal triad is best achieved by the use of damage control resuscitation, also known as hemostatic resuscitation. Hemostatic resuscitation is achieved by transfusing either FWB or component therapy in a 1:1:1 ratio, which mirrors the constituents of FWB. Key concepts of this process and evidence-based treatment are discussed next.

Acidosis

Metabolic acidosis in trauma is defined as a body pH less than 7.35. It results from prolonged hypoperfusion after trauma leading to anaerobic metabolism and the subsequent development of lactic acidosis. Acidosis may depress myocardial contractility and reduce cardiac output. Metabolic acidosis perpetuates further bleeding because of the inactivation of coagulation factors in acidic environments.[2]

Hypothermia

Defined as an abnormally low body temperature, less than 35°C, hypothermia leads to a slowing of physiologic activity. With trauma, hypothermia represents the cumulative effects of severe exsanguinating injury, resuscitative attempts, and exposure during surgery. During severe hemorrhage, the body loses the intrinsic ability to generate heat, known as thermogenesis, because of tissue hypoperfusion and reduced oxygen delivery to the tissues. Hypothermia compounds the lethal triad by inhibiting coagulation factors, promoting platelets dysfunction and fibrinolysis, contributing to further bleeding.[2]

Coagulopathy

Coagulopathy is defined as a disease or condition affecting the blood's ability to coagulate. It occurs after traumatic injuries because the delicate balance between hemostasis and fibrinolysis is disturbed, leading to significant coagulopathy.[12] Every aspect of coagulation is affected during massive fluid resuscitation as hemodilution exacerbates underlying coagulopathy and worsens acidosis leading to further ongoing blood loss.[2]

Fresh Whole Blood Transfusion

Transfusion of whole blood taken from a donor and given immediately to the patient with life-threatening hemorrhage, FWB transfusion is ideally type-specific, which signifies the donor is the same blood type as the recipient.[13]

1:1:1 Component Therapy

This refers to transfusion of blood components in a 1:1:1 ratio of packed RBCs (pRBCs), FFP, and platelets. A caveat of component therapy is platelets are generally not given until 4 to 6 U of red cells and plasma have been given. One unit of apheresis platelets is equivalent to a six-pack of pooled platelets.[14]

Nonhemostatic Resuscitation

Conventional hemorrhage resuscitation consists of crystalloid therapy to treat hypotension and pRBCs to increase oxygen carrying ability. In hemorrhagic shock, massive transfusion of stored pRBCs and crystalloid worsens metabolic acidosis and coagulopathy and leads to further bleeding by exacerbating the lethal triad.[15]

Hemostatic Resuscitation

The early use of whole blood or combined replacement of blood products in a 1:1:1 ratio as the primary resuscitation strategy aims to prevent dilutional coagulopathy and treat the intrinsic, or acute coagulopathy of trauma, through the replacement of each blood component in the same ratio as it is lost through hemorrhage.[3,16]

ACUTE COAGULOPATHY OF TRAUMA

Although coagulopathy in trauma is treatable, it has been implicated as the cause of almost half of hemorrhagic deaths in trauma patients.[16,17] Earlier theories illustrating the lethal triad presented as acidosis and hypothermia in response to hemorrhagic shock with coagulopathy developing later have been refuted, and evidence now suggests coagulopathy occurs immediately after trauma.[18] Other theories existed that advocated for damage control surgery, such as abbreviated laparotomy to stop bleeding, which would in turn avoid coagulopathy. However, as early as 1992, Burch and colleagues[19] in a retrospective study of 200 bleeding trauma patients reported more than half the patients died within the first 2 hours of resuscitation after abbreviated laparotomy (damage control surgery), suggesting simple correction of the source of bleeding did not halt exsanguination. Schreiber[10] conducted a similar study of damage control surgery to mitigate the effects of the lethal triad and found mortality rates decreased. However, the study concluded two important points. Improved damage control techniques affected better outcomes and the authors emphasized the requirement for early and aggressive blood product replacement with FFP, platelets, and cryoprecipitate. This study also suggested tissue factor exposure secondary to trauma results in activation of the coagulation cascade and consumption of coagulation factors.

MacLeod and colleagues[20] further supported the theory of acute coagulopathy with a review of prospective data collected on trauma patients presenting to a level I trauma center. Prothrombin time (PT), partial thromboplastin time (PTT), and platelet count were analyzed to determine whether coagulopathy is a predictor of mortality. They found early coagulopathy to be prevalent in 28% of patients on arrival to the trauma bay and that coagulopathy, early after trauma, is an independent predictor of mortality even in the presence of other risk factors. An initial abnormal PT increases the adjusted odds of dying by 35% and an initial abnormal PTT increases the adjusted odds of dying by 326%.[20] Holcomb and colleagues[21] stressed the importance of addressing the early coagulopathy of trauma because at the time the lethal triad is present in trauma patients, death is imminent. Conventional resuscitation has no place in traumatic hemorrhage and neglects direct treatment of coagulopathy, whereas what the authors describe as damage control resuscitation addresses the lethal triad on admission to the trauma bay thereby increasing survival.

Niles and colleagues[12] studied combat casualties, retrospectively, who required blood transfusion in a single combat hospital September 2003 to December 2004. Coagulation status, pH, base deficit, and temperature were compared on arrival according to injury severity score (ISS), injury patterns, and mortality. The study reported acute or early coagulopathy of trauma was rapidly diagnosed in the emergency department and was present in more than 33% of combat casualties who received transfusion. Coagulopathy was also independent of hypothermia but strongly correlated with acidosis and ISS. Injury severity was associated with mortality. The authors concluded early diagnosis and treatment of acute coagulopathy of trauma may improve outcomes.

Dries[22] studied patients who received massive transfusion with administration of plasma and platelets in a ratio equivalent to pRBCs (1:1:1). This study stimulated recognition of early coagulopathy occurring soon after injury; however, very little prospective data exist in this area. The authors reported early coagulopathy occurs in 25% of patients with large-volume tissue injuries and that early and aggressive administration of blood component therapy may reduce the overall amount of blood products. Thromboelastography provides real-time assessment of coagulation, whereas coagulation values lag behind (PT, PTT, and international normalized ratio). Floccard and colleagues[23] further supported the theory of early coagulopathy with their study of 45 trauma patients who had coagulation studies drawn on-scene and upon hospital admission. At the scene of the trauma, coagulation status was found to be abnormal in 56% of patients and protein C activities were decreased. On hospital admission coagulation status was abnormal in 60% of patients. PT, PTT, international normalized ratio, and protein activity were used to determine coagulopathy.

The existence of acute coagulopathy of trauma is supported in the literature, and may be explained in various ways. Much of the evidence suggests coagulopathy just after trauma results from a disruption of the delicate balance between hemostasis and fibrinolysis along with suggested activation of the protein C pathways.[16] Although the exact mechanism of the acute coagulopathy of trauma is currently unknown, it occurs frequently and is associated with increased mortality after hemorrhage.[12]

DEVELOPMENT OF MASSIVE TRANSFUSION PROTOCOLS

Early recognition of massive hemorrhage with immediate initiation of hemostatic massive transfusion therapy treats the acute coagulopathy of trauma and improves survival.[18] Polytrauma, associated with life-threatening hemorrhage, requires massive transfusion. Massive transfusion is defined by most trauma experts as the administration of more than 10 U of blood in a 24-hour period or greater than or equal to 5 U of blood in the first 4 hours.[8,14,24]

The administration of massive transfusion in the form of hemostatic resuscitation requires transfusing a deliberate ratio of components similar to the constituents of whole blood. Hemostatic resuscitation is accomplished by administering all blood components lost during traumatic hemorrhage in a ratio of 1:1:1 (pRBC/FFP/platelets) stored blood components or by giving warmed FWB.[6] A caveat of 1:1:1 component therapy is platelets are generally not given until 4 to 6 U of pRBCs and FFP have been given. One unit of apheresis platelets is equivalent to a six-pack of pooled platelets.[14] FWB transfusion is provided by taking whole blood from a donor and administering it immediately to the patient with life-threatening hemorrhage. FWB is ideally type-specific, which signifies the donor is the same blood type as the recipient.[13] Massive transfusion protocols (MTP) in the civilian sector, still early in their practice infancy, are based on the delivery of 1:1:1 component ratios, not FWB.

Until recently there has been little evidence to guide blood component usage during massive transfusion. New data from recent wars have driven an evolution of opinion in military and civilian trauma communities for the optimal resuscitative approach to life-threatening hemorrhage, prompting transfusion medicine to move from reactive treatment with crystalloid and pRBC therapy to use of a standardized MTP.[3,25] The implementation of MTPs recommending 1:1:1 transfusion provides standardization among trauma centers and promotes rapid execution of the most effective resuscitation therapies while reducing blood product waste.[26,27] Unfortunately, in reality, there is significant regional and institutional variability in the treatment of coagulopathy and surprisingly few institutions have MTPs in place.[28] The American Society of Anesthesiologists updated practice guidelines for perioperative blood management in February 2015, which is written by a task force and largely relied on expert opinion for guidance. For hemorrhagic bleeding, however, the guideline recommends the use of an institutional MTP.[29] There are numerous citations in literature regarding implementation and modification of existing MTPs; along with anecdotal reports and national meeting discussions, it is clear that more and more centers have MTPs and most embrace the tenants of damage control resuscitation.[30,31]

IMPLICATIONS FOR FRESH WHOLE BLOOD TRANSFUSION

Use of FWB is primarily described in the military literature for treatment of traumatic hemorrhage because it is associated with halting the lethal triad and improving outcomes. It is likely that FWB may also be used to treat hemorrhage not associated with trauma, such as massive bleeding associated with surgical misadventure or obstetric emergencies. For example, during obstetric emergencies improved availability of blood transfusions has dramatically reduced maternal mortality during the twentieth century; yet obstetric hemorrhage still remains a leading cause of maternal death. In 2005, hemorrhage was the third leading cause of maternal death in the United States because of obstetric factors.[32] The common causes of maternal death from hemorrhage include placental abruption, retained placenta, uterine rupture, uterine atony, and placental implantation disorders. Pregnancy emergencies such as these demand obstetric care including the capability of prompt administration of blood products.

A further benefit to FWB transfusion used to treat acute coagulopathy in hemorrhagic trauma is the observed decrease in overall blood product use. In 2005, reported trauma involving blood loss of greater than 40% blood volume signified irreversible hemorrhagic shock and death in the face of massive transfusion, which depletes blood banks and costs more than $50,000 per patient.[33] The overall reduction of blood product administration is not only important from a cost standpoint, but also for the potential reduction in morbidity among survivors. Numerous authors have demonstrated an increase in acute lung injury, acute respiratory distress syndrome, and multiple system organ failure with massive transfusion with multiple blood components.[34–37] By minimizing hemorrhage early and decreasing overall blood product use, the incidence and severity of these morbidities may also be reduced.[38]

ADVANTAGES OF FRESH WHOLE BLOOD OVER COMPONENT THERAPY

A search of the literature reveals no previous studies comparing outcomes for patients transfused with FWB compared with component therapy administered in civilian trauma settings in any population because it is almost exclusively used in combat operations.[6] Recent studies have shown 1:1:1 blood component and/or FWB use is associated with increased survival rates approaching 96%, which is a reversal from previous studies that reported 98% mortality after conventional resuscitation.[2,6,18] Conventional component therapy does not include the administration of plasma, platelets, and cryoprecipitate until late in the resuscitation when coagulation studies indicate the need for clotting factors and platelets replacement. This is primarily because the goal of conventional resuscitation is to treat late occurring coagulopathy caused by acidosis and hypothermia. Blood product amounts administered during conventional component therapy often fall significantly below what is needed to address the complex coagulopathy related to dilution, consumption, and fibrinolysis and worsen the effects of the lethal triad.[25] Conventional component therapy is now referred to in the literature as nonhemostatic resuscitation and is independently associated with uncontrolled bleeding, which increases the volume of blood lost in uncontrolled hemorrhage, involves massive amounts of blood products,[26] and lowers survival rates.[14]

Survival rates are much higher when hemostatic resuscitation techniques are administered according to MTP. In fact, the highest survival rates are associated with the administration of FWB (96%) compared with 1:1:1 component therapy (82%) alone.[6] This suggests FWB is superior to 1:1:1 component therapy in treating massive hemorrhage.

Although a single unit of warm FWB (500 mL) may be roughly equivalent in volume to 1:1:1 component therapy (680 mL), FWB has several advantages over component therapy. First, FWB does not need to be warmed because it is immediately administered after collection from the donor. Second, it has a higher concentration of RBCs and platelets, contains 100% of original clotting factors, and has double the fibrinogen.[39] These qualities of FWB make it more effective in reversing coagulopathy and transporting oxygen. In addition, warm FWB has fewer anticoagulants in contrast to component blood, which has anticoagulant preservative additives; pRBCs are also at $0°C$ to prolong shelf life and require blood warmer technology, not always available far forward. Cold, old blood with added anticoagulants worsens coagulopathy of trauma. The use of FWB has been shown clinically to improve the ability of the blood to clot, reverse dilutional coagulopathy, and provide a hemostatic effect comparable with 10 U of platelets.[39]

Although advocating a FWB MTP may seem radical, the evidence supporting current transfusion practices is generally underwhelming. The literature from the war zone suggests FWB is more efficient than stored 1:1:1 component therapy at correcting acute coagulopathy and reversing hemorrhagic shock in war casualties while also minimizing the adverse effects of transfusion storage lesions from older RBCs.[6] Strandenes and colleagues[40] emphasized the need for FWB collection mechanisms, field blood banks, to support the special operators during high-risk missions on the far forward battlefield. With the previous experiences of exsanguination of Special Forces soldiers, FWB was used because stored blood components are relatively unavailable. Additionally, it is anticipated the number of transfusions necessary to reverse the lethal triad will be reduced with the use of FWB.[25]

INFECTIOUS DISEASE TESTING

The use of FWB in the military includes a rapid test for infectious disease, which requires only 5 hours of testing. However, the rapid test is not approved by the Food and Drug Administration and hinders the proliferation of FWB use in civilian trauma.[6] The literature supports the need for further research on a scientific level to determine the mechanisms underlying survival, and in the systems management level to ensure compliance with infectious disease testing, and the feasibility of FWB use in nonwartime settings.[25] As a result of the potential survival benefits of FWB, efforts are being made to improve the safety of the whole blood donor pool, which includes human immunodeficiency virus and hepatitis B and C screening for all US military personnel before deployment.[6] Development of infectious disease testing methods should instead be emphasized to minimize the risk for transmission and make FWB more widely available for the severe trauma patients who need it.

SUMMARY

Severe traumatic injury is a public health care problem of modern society. Trauma results in the death of more than 5 million people annually worldwide and this number is expected to increase to more than 8 million by 2020.[41] The number of deaths from injury has not declined for more than a decade despite efforts to affect its prevention.[42] Improvement in survival outcomes for patients requiring massive transfusion is of utmost importance to military and civilian trauma communities. Damage control surgery following trauma has developed as a major advance in surgical practice over the past 30 years.[43] Rapid progress has recently been made with damage control resuscitation measures because of the severity of injured casualties from the military experiences in the Middle East; translational research is needed to standardize and better integrate these new principles of hemostatic damage control resuscitation into civilian trauma clinical practice. The earlier these protocols are instituted, the higher the chances for survival. Unfortunately, most trauma centers rely on clinical judgment alone to institute MTP.[44] Although management of hemorrhage focuses on control of blood loss and replacement of circulating volume, best practices related to transfusion medicine have yet to be established.[45] Finally, Bawazeer and colleagues,[46] reported there exists little specific literature in regard to standardized resuscitation methods and the absence of clear recommendations may lead to poor compliance to institutional MTPs.

Conventional component therapy was chosen over whole blood transfusion in the 1970s with little evidence to support the change in practice and without regard to life-threatening hemorrhage management. Recent evidence suggests FWB is superior to 1:1:1 component therapy in reversing the lethal triad of hemorrhage and ultimately increasing survival rates; studies also suggest overall blood use is less with FWB transfusion. Unfortunately, most of the evidence that exists is a result of retrospective examination of the successful treatment of polytrauma in Iraq and Afghanistan. It is also well documented that the shelf life of blood components was extended by the US military during the recent wars to assist with blood stores. However, extended storage of blood components has been shown to worsen the clinical picture of severe hemorrhage because of storage lesions that occur in blood after 14 days. Instead increased survival after transfusion of FWB rich in platelets and clotting factors may be caused by the effective reversal the acute coagulopathy of trauma.

In any civilian disaster the need for FWB is a potentially life-saving mechanism. The September 11, 2001 experience in New York City is an excellent illustration of how FWB can be used. If a significant proportion of those who had been killed during the World Trade Center collapse had instead survived and required massive transfusion, blood component stores would have been depleted rapidly. At the time transport into the region, particularly air transport, was blocked. Without available component therapy, the use of FWB in this kind of extreme circumstance would potentially have been recognized.[47] The use of whole blood in such disaster circumstances is ideal because it is immediately available, it does not require storage or warming, and is life-saving as demonstrated in recent studies where it has been at least equivalent to or more effective than 1:1:1 component therapy. It has also been shown to be associated with a decreased use of all blood products required for massive transfusion in austere environments.

Although the use of FWB is primarily described in the military literature for treatment of traumatic hemorrhage, its benefits of halting the lethal triad and improving survival outcomes also increase desirability within the civilian populations. It is likely that FWB may also be used to treat hemorrhage not associated with trauma, such as massive bleeding associated with surgical misadventure or obstetric emergencies. Effective hemostatic resuscitation tailored to the physiologic condition of patients with life-threatening hemorrhage could potentially eradicate death by exsanguination related to severe trauma or any other coagulopathy while also decreasing overall use of blood products.

REFERENCES

1. Curry N, Hopewell S, Doree C, et al. The acute management of trauma hemorrhage: a systematic review of randomized controlled trials. Crit Care 2011; 15:R92.
2. Jaunoo SS, Harji DP. Damage control surgery. Int J Surg 2009;7:110–3.
3. Holcomb JB, Spinella PC. Optimal use of blood in trauma patients. Biologicals 2010;38(1):72.
4. Schrager JJ, Branson RD, Johannigman JA. Lessons from the tip of the spear: medical advancements from Iraq and Afghanistan. Respir Care 2012;57(8): 1305–13.
5. Spahn DR, Rossaint R. Coagulopathy and blood component transfusion in trauma. Br J Anaesth 2005;95(2):130–9.
6. Spinella PC, Perkins JG, Grathwohl KW, et al. Warm fresh whole blood is independently associated with improved survival for patients with combat-related traumatic injuries. J Trauma 2009;66(4):S69–76.
7. Scalea TM. Hemostatic resuscitation for acute traumatic coagulopathy. Scand J Trauma Resusc Emerg Med 2011;19(2):1–2.
8. Holcomb JB. Damage control resuscitation. J Trauma 2007;62:S36–7.
9. Nessen SC, Eastridge BJ, Cronk D, et al. Fresh whole blood use by forward surgical teams in Afghanistan is associated with improved survival compared to CT without platelets. Transfusion 2013;53(S1):107S–13S.
10. Schreiber MA. Damage control surgery. Crit Care Clin 2004;20:101–18.
11. Mikhail, Judy. The trauma triad of death: hypothermia, acidosis, and coagulopathy. AACN Advanced Critical Care 1999;10(1):85–94.
12. Niles SE, McLaughlin DF, Perkins JG, et al. Increased mortality associated with the early coagulopathy of trauma in combat casualties. J Trauma 2008;64(6): 1459–65.
13. Kauvar DS, Holcomb JB, Norris GC, et al. Fresh whole blood transfusion: a controversial military practice. J Trauma 2006;61(1):181–4.
14. Borgman MA, Spinella PC, Perkins JG, et al. Ratio of blood products transfused affects mortality in patients receiving massive transfusions at a combat support hospital. J Trauma 2007;63:805–13.
15. Holcomb JB, Wade CE, Michalek JE, et al. Increased plasma and platelet to red blood cell rations improves outcome in 466 massively transfused civilian trauma patients. Ann Surg 2008;248(3):447–58.
16. Duchesne JC, McSwain NE, Cotton BA, et al. Damage control resuscitation: the new face of damage control. J Trauma 2010;69(4):976–90.
17. Duchesne JC, Hunt JP, Wahl G, et al. Review of current blood transfusions strategies in a mature level I trauma center: were we wrong for the last 60 years? J Trauma 2008;65(2):272–8.
18. Holcomb JB, Del Junco DJ, Fox EE, et al. The prospective, observational, multicenter major trauma transfusion (PROMMTT) study. Arch Surg 2012. http://dx.doi.org/10.1001/2013.jamasurg.387.
19. Burch JM, Ortiz VB, Richardson RJ, et al. Abbreviated laparotomy and planned reoperation for critically injured patients. Ann Surg 1992;215(5): 476–83.
20. MacLeod JB, Lynn M, McKenney MG, et al. Early coagulopathy predicts mortality in trauma. J Trauma 2003;55(1):39–44.
21. Holcomb JB, Jenkins D, Rhee P, et al. Damage control resuscitation: directly addressing the early coagulopathy of trauma. J Trauma 2007;62(2):307–10.

22. Dries DJ. The contemporary role of blood products and components used in trauma resuscitation. Scand J Trauma Resusc Emerg Med 2010;18(63):34.
23. Floccard B, Rugeri L, Faure A, et al. Early coagulopathy in trauma patients: an on-scene and hospital admission study. Injury 2012;43(1):26–32.
24. Mitra B, Mori A, Cameron PA, et al. Fresh frozen plasma (FFP) use during massive blood transfusion in trauma resuscitation. Injury 2010;41(1):35–9.
25. Young PP, Cotton BA, Goodnough LT. Massive transfusion protocols for patients with substantial hemorrhage. Transfus Med Rev 2011;25(4):293–303.
26. Hannon T. Trauma blood management: avoiding the collateral damage of trauma resuscitation protocols. Hematology 2010;2010(1):463–4.
27. Holcomb JB. Traditional transfusion practices are changing. Crit Care 2010; 14(3):162.
28. Napolitano LM. Guideline compliance in trauma: evidence-based protocols to improve trauma outcomes?*. Crit Care Med 2012;40(3):990–2.
29. American Society of Anesthesiologists Task Force on Perioperative Blood Management. Practice guidelines for perioperative blood management: an updated report by the American Society of Anesthesiologists task force on perioperative blood management*. Anesthesiology 2015;122(2):241–75.
30. Cohen MJ. Towards hemostatic resuscitation: the changing understanding of acute traumatic biology, massive bleeding, and damage-control resuscitation. Surg Clin North Am 2012;92(4):877–91.
31. Cotton BA, Podbielski J, Camp E, et al. A randomized controlled pilot trial of modified whole blood versus component therapy in severely injured patients requiring large volume transfusions. Ann Surg 2013;258(4):527–33.
32. Alexander JM, Sarode R, McIntire DD, et al. Whole blood in the management of hypovolemia due to obstetric hemorrhage. Obstet Gynecol 2009;113(6): 1320–6.
33. Criddle LM, Eldredge DH, Walker J. Variables predicting trauma patient survival following massive transfusion. J Emerg Nurs 2005;31:236–42.
34. Bux J. Transfusion-related acute lung injury (TRALI): a serious adverse event of blood transfusion. Vox Sang 2005;89(1):1–10.
35. Marik PE, Corwin HL. Acute lung injury following blood transfusion: expanding the definition. Crit Care Med 2008;36(11):3080–4.
36. Robinson WP III, Ahn J, Stiffler A, et al. Blood transfusion is an independent predictor of increased mortality in nonoperatively managed blunt hepatic and splenic injuries. J Trauma 2005;58(3):437–45.
37. Watson GA, Sperry JL, Rosengart MR, et al. Fresh frozen plasma is independently associated with a higher risk of multiple organ failure and acute respiratory distress syndrome. J Trauma 2009;67(2):221–30.
38. Cotton BA, Gunter OL, Isbell J, et al. Damage control hematology: the impact of a trauma exsanguination protocol on survival and blood product utilization. J Trauma 2008;64(5):1177–83.
39. Bowling F, Pennardt A. The use of fresh whole blood transfusions by the SOF medic for hemostatic resuscitation in the austere environment. J Spec Oper Med 2010;10(3):25–35.
40. Strandenes G, Cap AP, Cacic D, et al. Blood Far Forward—a whole blood research and training program for austere environments. Transfusion 2013; 53(S1):124S–30S.
41. Spahn DR, Bouillon B, Cerny V, et al. Management of bleeding and coagulopathy following major trauma: an updated European guideline. Crit Care 2013; 17(2):R76.

42. Shaz BH, Dente CJ, Harris RS, et al. Transfusion management of trauma patients. Anesth Analg 2009;108(6):1760.
43. Dadhwal US, Pathak N. Damage control philosophy in polytrauma. Med J Armed Forces India 2010;66(4):347–9.
44. Nunez TC, Voskresensky IV, Dossett LA, et al. Early prediction of massive transfusion in trauma: simple as ABC (assessment of blood consumption)? J Trauma 2009;66(2):346–52.
45. Jones AR, Frazier SK. Increased mortality in adult trauma patients transfused with blood components compared with whole blood. J Trauma Nurs 2014;21(1):22.
46. Bawazeer M, Ahmed N, Izadi H, et al. Compliance with a massive transfusion protocol (MTP) impacts patient outcome. Injury 2015;46(1):21–8.
47. Repine TB, Perkins JG, Kauvar DS, et al. The use of fresh whole blood in massive transfusion. J Trauma 2006;60:S59–69.

Pain and Agitation Management in Critically Ill Patients

Julie Stephens, PharmD, BCPS[a],*, Michael Wright, PharmD, BCPS[b]

KEYWORDS

- Agitation • Sedation • Pharmacotherapy • Pain • Analgosedation • Opioid

KEY POINTS

- Vital signs alone should not be used to assess pain; well-validated behavioral pain scales are most appropriate for pain assessment in the intensive care unit.
- Opiate selection should be based on the patient's opiate tolerance and the pharmacokinetic properties of the medication.
- All sedation should be titrated to light sedation or patients should receive a daily spontaneous awakening trial.
- Analgosedation is recommended for the treatment of agitation. If patients require further sedation, it is recommended to add a nonbenzodiazepine sedative, such as propofol or dexmedetomidine.

INTRODUCTION

Since 1995, groups such as the American College of Critical Care Medicine, the Society of Critical Care Medicine, the American Society of Health-System Pharmacists, and others have been dedicated to improving the treatment of pain and agitation in intensive care unit (ICU) patients.[1-3] The most recent set of guidelines, developed by a multidisciplinary panel, focused on the prevention and treatment of pain, agitation, and delirium in critically ill patients. The guidelines contain evidence-based recommendations published through December 2010, as an update to the guidelines published in 2002. These guidelines are referenced frequently as they provide the standard of care for critically ill patients.[1,2]

Disclosure Statement: The authors have nothing to disclose.
[a] Department of Pharmacy Practice, Lipscomb University College of Pharmacy, One University Park Drive, Nashville, TN 37204, USA; [b] Department of Pharmacy, Williamson Medical Center, 4321 Carothers Parkway, Franklin, TN 37067, USA
* Corresponding author.
E-mail address: Julie.wilbeck@Lipscomb.edu

Nurs Clin N Am 51 (2016) 95–106
http://dx.doi.org/10.1016/j.cnur.2015.11.002   nursing.theclinics.com

PAIN IN THE INTENSIVE CARE UNIT

It is common for critically ill patients to experience pain at some point during their ICU stay. This pain could be related to invasive procedures, external lines and tubes, extensive surgery, trauma, or chronic underlying conditions. Most patients who have been intubated recall some pain associated with the endotracheal tube.[4] Most cardiac surgery patients state pain as a common traumatic memory of their ICU visit.[5] In medical and surgical ICUs, the incidence of pain is 50% or higher.[6,7]

The subjective nature of pain is a significant obstacle in the development of quality pain assessment tools. It is recommended that vital signs alone not be used to assess pain in ICU patients.[8–11] However, vital signs could be used as impetus for further assessment. Patient self-reporting of pain has been considered the gold standard pain assessment, but this may not be feasible in all ICU patients. In patients who are unable to self-report pain, one should consider looking at the patients' behaviors as an indicator of pain. Several behavioral pain scales have been created over the past few years. However, it is difficult to determine their applicability to the ICU population. Studies have demonstrated that implementation of a behavioral pain scale in the ICU improves clinical outcomes, such as decreasing length of stay and days of mechanical ventilation.[12,13] The most suitable behavioral pain scales for use in ICU patients are the Critical-Care Pain Observation Tool and the Behavioral Pain Scale.[8,11,14,15] These pain scales are most appropriate for adult patients with intact motor function who are unable to self-report pain.

TREATMENT OF PAIN

The optimal agent for the treatment of pain in the ICU should be based on individual patient characteristics and response. When selecting an analgesic, careful consideration should be given to the pharmacokinetic and pharmacodynamic properties of all available agents. The mainstays of therapy in the ICU are fentanyl, hydromorphone, morphine, and methadone. These agents belong to a class of medications called opioids and primarily exert their mechanism of action by agonizing μ receptor subtypes, which, in turn, blunts the emotional response to pain. Respiratory depression and decreased gastrointestinal motility are common adverse effects of opioid analgesics.[16–18] With the exception of ketamine, nonopiate analgesics have limited efficacy data for non-neuropathic pain in the ICU setting, so their use is limited (**Table 1**).

Fentanyl

Fentanyl is a potent μ receptor agonist used for the management of pain in acute care and outpatient settings. It has poor enteral bioavailability, so it is typically administered via transmucosal, intravenous (IV), and transdermal routes. The onset of IV fentanyl is approximately 1 to 2 minutes, and the elimination half-life is around 2 to 4 hours. However, fentanyl has a short duration of action lasting approximately 0.5 to 1.0 hour after IV administration. The short duration of action is due to fentanyl being very lipophilic and redistributing rapidly after administration. Fentanyl is entirely eliminated via hepatic metabolism, specifically cytochrome P450 (CYP) 3A4, 3A5, and N-dealkylation, producing no active metabolites. The typical infusion dosage is 0.7 to 10.0 mcg/kg/h for mechanically ventilated patients. Fentanyl is less likely than morphine to induce histamine release, making it a more desirable agent in patients exhibiting hemodynamic instability.[3,19,20] Fentanyl's short duration of action, rapid onset, and lack of active metabolites make it an excellent analgesic for a wide range of critically ill patients.

Table 1
Opiate analgesics

Opiates	MOA	Onset	Half-life (h)	Accumulation	Typical Adult Dosage (IV)	Adverse Effects
Fentanyl	μ Agonist	1–2 min	2–4	Decreased metabolism in hepatic failure	0.7–10.0 mcg/kg/h	Hypotension, constipation, accumulation with hepatic impairment
Hydromorphone	μ Agonist	5–15 min	2–3	Decreased metabolism in hepatic failure	0.5–3.0 mg/h	Hypotension, constipation
Morphine	μ Agonist	5–10 min	3–4	Decreased metabolism in hepatic failure; active metabolite accumulation in renal failure	2–30 mg/h	Hypotension, constipation
Methadone	μ Agonist, NMDA antagonist	1–3 d	15–60	Decreased metabolism in hepatic failure	2.5–10.0 mg q8–12 h	Constipation, QTc prolongation

Abbreviations: GABA, γ-aminobutyric acid; MOA, mechanism of action; NMDA, N-methyl-ᴅ-aspartate; QTc, Q-T interval corrected.
Data from Refs. [19,20,25]

Hydromorphone

Hydromorphone is another potent μ receptor agonist used for the management of pain in the acute care setting. It has an oral bioavailability of 24%, and is typically administered intravenously. The onset of IV hydromorphone is approximately 5 to 15 minutes, and the elimination half-life is approximately 2 to 3 hours. Hydromorphone is eliminated via extensive hepatic metabolism, specifically glucuronidation, producing no active metabolites. The typical infusion dosage is 0.5 to 3.0 mg/h for mechanically ventilated patients. Hydromorphone is less likely than morphine to induce histamine release, making it a more desirable agent in patients exhibiting hemodynamic instability. The increased potency of hydromorphone at the μ receptor is a cause for greater concern due to respiratory depression. Respiratory depression is relatively uncommon as long as the infusion is titrated slowly or intermittent doses are given at reasonable intervals, such as every 2 to 3 hours. Hydromorphone's short duration of action, potency, and lack of active metabolites make it an excellent analgesic for critically ill patients who are tolerant to fentanyl or morphine, regardless of hemodynamic stability.

Morphine

Morphine is a μ receptor agonist used for the management of pain in the acute care and outpatient settings. It has an oral bioavailability of 17% to 33% and is administered via oral, subcutaneous, and IV routes. The onset of IV morphine is approximately 5 to 10 minutes, and the elimination half-life is approximately 3 to 4 hours. Morphine is eliminated via hepatic metabolism, specifically glucuronidation, producing 2 active metabolites. The active metabolites undergo renal elimination, making this agent's elimination somewhat unpredictable in a patient with significant renal impairment. The typical infusion dosage is 2 to 30 mg/h for mechanically ventilated patients, but this depends heavily on the patient's prior exposure to opiates. It is common for morphine to induce histamine release causing hypotension and pruritus, making this agent much less desirable in patients exhibiting hemodynamic instability.[3,19] Morphine's longer duration of action, relatively low potency, and active metabolites make it reasonable choice for critically ill patients who are opiate naïve and hemodynamically stable with good renal function.

Methadone

Methadone is a μ receptor agonist and an N-methyl-D-aspartate (NMDA) receptor antagonist used for the management of pain in the acute care and outpatient settings. The NMDA receptor activity may slow the development of opiate tolerance. It has an oral bioavailability of greater than 36% and is administered via oral and IV routes. The onset of IV methadone is approximately 15 minutes; however, the peak analgesic effect occurs between days 3 and 5. Therefore, the dose should not be increased any more frequently than every 3 days. The elimination half-life is biphasic with an initial phase of 12 to 24 hours and a secondary phase of 55 hours. Methadone is eliminated via extensive hepatic metabolism, producing one active metabolite. Methadone is administered in an intermittent dosing fashion with the typical dosage ranging from 2.5 to 10 mg every 8 to 12 hours for mechanically ventilated patients, but this depends heavily on patients' prior exposure to opiates. Patients who are tolerant to opiates may require less methadone than would be expected based on a simple dose-equivalent conversion. It is very well established that methadone prolongs the Q-T interval corrected (QTc). Monitoring the QTc while on methadone is recommended. The risks versus benefits of methadone should be evaluated if the QTc exceeds 500 milliseconds because of the high risk of torsades de pointes.[3,19,25] The NMDA receptor antagonism makes methadone a good alternative for patients who are rapidly developing opiate tolerance or may have been taking methadone before admission.

Ketamine

Ketamine is an NMDA receptor antagonist used to induce dissociative anesthesia as well as pain management in the acute care setting. It has an oral bioavailability of 16% and is administered via IV and intramuscular routes. The onset of IV ketamine is approximately 10 to 15 minutes, and the elimination half-life is approximately 2 to 3 hours. Ketamine is eliminated via hepatic metabolism, specifically the N-demethylation via CYP system producing one active metabolite. The recommended infusion dosage is 0.05 to 0.4 mg/kg/h as an adjunctive agent in patients receiving an opiate while undergoing mechanical ventilation. Commonly reported adverse effects of ketamine include hypertension, tachycardia, and increased intracranial pressure, making this agent less than ideal for patients with an aortic dissection, stroke, traumatic brain injury, or clinically significant hypertension. Emergence reactions, which consist of auditory and visual hallucinations, disorientation, and vivid dreams, are common with ketamine use. Ketamine alone and in combination with opiates often causes respiratory depression and should be discontinued during daily awakening periods. Ketamine should not be considered the first line for analgesia in most critically ill adults.[19,26] Ketamine's unique mechanism of action makes it a good choice for patients with a high degree of opioid tolerance.

NEUROPATHIC PAIN
Gabapentin

Gabapentin binds to voltage-gated calcium channels throughout the brain and is commonly used to treat neuropathic pain and partial onset seizures. Gabapentin in combination with opiates has shown greater efficacy than carbamazepine for the treatment of neuropathic pain in the critically ill.[27] It is only available in oral formulations and administered via enteral routes. Gabapentin undergoes renal elimination and has a half-life of 5 to 7 hours. The recommended starting dosage is 100 mg 3 times daily, with a maintenance dose of 900 to 3600 mg in 3 divided doses. Dose adjustment is required in patients with renal insufficiency. The medication is generally well tolerated but should not be discontinued abruptly as this may increase risk of seizures. The most common adverse effects include sedation, confusion, and ataxia.[3,28]

Carbamazepine

Carbamazepine is a neural sodium channel antagonist used to treat partial or generalized tonic-clonic seizures as well as neuropathic pain. Carbamazepine in combination with opiates has shown significantly greater efficacy than placebo for the treatment of neuropathic pain in the critically ill.[27] It is only available in oral formulations. Carbamazepine is eliminated via hepatic metabolism, specifically CYP 3A4, and is an auto-inducer. The initial half-life is 25 to 65 hours and then decreases to 5 to 7 hours approximately 3 to 5 weeks after initiation. The recommended starting dosage is 100 mg twice daily, with a maintenance dosage of 100 to 200 mg every 6 hours. A 25% dose reduction is recommended in patients with end-stage renal disease. Carbamazepine has been associated with several serious adverse events, including agranulocytosis, toxic epidermal necrolysis, Stevens-Johnson syndrome, and hyponatremia. Most common adverse effects include sedation, confusion, blurred vision, and ataxia.[3,19,28]

SEDATION

Agitation and anxiety are common problems in the ICU. Patients often experience pain, confusion, delirium, hypoxia, and substance withdrawal, among other unpleasant factors while in the ICU. Before administering pharmacologic sedatives, treatment of the underlying issue should first be attempted. If the underlying issue cannot be resolved or adequately controlled, then sedatives may be clinically indicated. Sedatives should typically be titrated to maintain a light level of sedation, whereby patients are still able to be aroused and perform purposeful movements. The use of light sedation has been shown to decrease mechanical ventilation time and ICU length of stay.[23]

LEVEL OF SEDATION

Balancing patients' sedation is important, as the patients' sedation goal must be achieved while minimizing the risk of adverse events. The purpose of sedation is to facilitate mechanical ventilation, alleviate anxiety and agitation, and to provide caregiver safety. Oversedation may lead to muscle atrophy, weakness, pneumonia, further ventilator dependence, and delirium. Patients should be routinely monitored for their depth and quality of sedation at least once every nursing shift. If sedation scales are to be used, the Richmond Agitation-Sedation Scale (RASS) **Table 2** and Riker Sedation-Agitation Scale (SAS) are the two guideline-recommended scales as they are considered the most reliable and valid for ICU patients. The two scales are similar and have the ability to not only discern between levels of sedation but also levels of agitation.[23]

Table 2 **Richmond Agitation-Sedation Scale**		
Score	Term	Description
+4	Combative	Overtly combative or violent, immediate danger to staff
+3	Very agitated	Pulls on or removes tube(s) or catheter(s) or exhibits aggressive behavior toward staff
+2	Agitated	Frequent nonpurposeful movement or patient-ventilator dys-synchrony
+1	Restless	Anxious or apprehensive but movements not aggressive or Vigorous
0	Alert and calm	
−1	Drowsy	Not fully alert, but has sustained (>10 seconds) awakening, with eye contact, to voice
−2	Light sedation	Briefly (<10 seconds) awakens with eye contact to voice
−3	Moderate sedation	Any movement (but no eye contact) to voice
−4	Deep sedation	No response to voice, but any movement to physical stimulation
−5	Unarousable	No response to voice or physical stimulation

Performed using a series of steps: observation of behaviors (score +4 to 0), followed (if necessary) by assessment of response to voice (score −1 to −3), followed (if necessary) by assessment of response to physical stimulation such as shaking shoulder and then rubbing sternum if no response to shaking shoulder (score −4 to −5).

Reprinted from Sessler CN, Gosnell MS, Grap MJ, et al. The Richmond Agitation–Sedation Scale. Am J Respir Crit Care Med;166(10):1338–44; with permission of the American Thoracic Society. Copyright © 2015 American Thoracic Society. *The American Journal of Respiratory and Critical Care Medicine* is an official journal of the American Thoracic Society.

One strategy, in addition to light sedation, is to perform a spontaneous awakening trial (SAT) as in Girard and colleagues.[29] SATs are daily interruptions of sedatives. All sedatives and analgesics that are used for sedation are discontinued. Any analgesics used for active pain are continued. Patients are then monitored by staff for awakening or signs of failure, which include anxiety, agitation, cardiac arrhythmias, or at least 2 signs of respiratory distress. These SATs when paired with spontaneous breathing trials have been shown to successfully decrease the time on the ventilator, decrease ICU and hospital length of stay, as well as shorten the duration of coma. The protocol also improved 1-year survival when compared with usual care. SATs lead to less over-sedation and also allow the practitioner to assess patients' underlying neurologic function on a daily basis.[29]

Deep sedation may still be indicated for some patients in the ICU. When deep sedation is achieved, patients are not able to be aroused. This sedation should be used when patients are receiving neuromuscular blocking agents and will be paralyzed or when patients exhibit poor ventilator compliance. The patients should be deeply sedated before a neuromuscular blocking agent is administered. The patients should also have an objective measure of brain function guiding sedation while receiving a neuromuscular blocker. While patients are chemically paralyzed, RASS or SAS assessments are unreliable. Examples of objective measures of brain function include bispectral index, auditory evoked potential measurement, and others.[23]

SEDATIVE AGENTS

When comparing the hypnotic sedatives, the guidelines recommend nonbenzodiazepine agents (eg, dexmedetomidine and propofol) over benzodiazepine agents.[23] In 2013, Fraser and colleagues published a meta-analysis reviewing randomized trials comparing nonbenzodiazepine regimens with benzodiazepine regimens. They reviewed 83 articles from 1996 and included 6 articles in the analysis. They found that use of a nonbenzodiazepine sedation was associated with a shorter ICU length of stay (1.65 days; 95% confidence interval [CI], 0.72–2.58; $P=.0005$). Nonbenzodiazepine regimens were also associated with shorter duration of mechanical ventilation (mean difference 1.9 days; 95% CI, 1.70–2.09; $P<.00001$). Risk of death was similar between the two regiments (relative risk, 0.98%; 95% CI, 0.76–1.27; $P=.94$). This data, along with smaller studies, emphasizes the importance of using nonbenzodiazepine sedation when feasible.[30] Careful considerations, such as comorbidities and duration of planned sedation, must also be taken into account when selecting a sedative agent (**Table 3**).

Dexmedetomidine

Dexmedetomidine is a selective alpha$_2$-adrenergic agonist with a Food and Drug Administration (FDA) indication for ICU sedation of mechanically ventilated patients for less than 24 hours and for procedural sedation of nonintubated patients.[21] Since the FDA approval of dexmedetomidine, several studies have demonstrated the use of infusions administered for longer than 24 hours and at dosages exceeding the approved 0.2 to 0.7 mcg/kg/h. Dosages of up to 1.5 mcg/kg/h have been shown to be safe and effective for ICU sedation. The benefits of dexmedetomidine include opioid-sparing effects, minimal effect on respiratory drive, increase in sleep-wave activity, and has the least risk of causing ICU delirium; patients are more easily aroused than those sedated on other medications.[31,32] Common side effects include hypotension and bradycardia. Additionally, similar to clonidine, patients may experience withdrawal with administration of prolonged dexmedetomidine. It is

Table 3
Sedative agents

Sedative (Brand)	MOA	Onset	Half-life	Accumulation	Typical Adult Dosage	Adverse Effects	Other Effects
Dexmedetomidine (Precedex)[1,21]	α_2 agonist	15 min	2 h	Decreased metabolism in hepatic failure	0.2–1.5 mcg/kg/min	Hypotension, bradycardia	Analgesic/opioid sparing, sympatholytic
Propofol (Diprivan)[1,22]	Receptor agonist: GABA$_A$, glycine, nicotinic, and M$_1$ muscarinic receptors	1–2 min	3–12 h (short-term use); 1–3 d (long-term use)	Increased accumulation with prolonged use	5–50 mcg/kg/min	Respiratory depression, hypotension, hypertriglyceridemia, acute pancreatitis, soy and egg allergic reactions	Hypnotic, anxiolytic, amnestic, antiemetic, anticonvulsant
Midazolam (Versed)[1,23]	GABA$_A$ agonist	1.5–2.5 min	1.4–2.4 h (up to 10 h in elderly)	Decreased metabolism in hepatic failure; accumulation in renal failure and with prolonged use; clearance decreases with age	0.03–0.2 mg/kg/h	Respiratory depression, hypotension, strong correlation with ICU delirium	Hypnotic, anxiolytic, amnestic, anticonvulsant
Lorazepam (Ativan)[1,24] *Note off-label use	GABA$_A$ agonist	15–20 min	14 ± 5 h	Decreased metabolism in hepatic failure; increased elimination half-life and duration of effect in renal failure; clearance decreases with age	0.01–0.1 mg/kg/h (max 10 mg/h)	Respiratory depression, hypotension, propylene glycol toxicity, strong correlation with ICU delirium	Hypnotic, anxiolytic, amnestic, anticonvulsant

recommended that patients be monitored for signs and symptoms of withdrawal if they have received dexmedetomidine for 7 days or longer. Dexmedetomidine withdrawal is treated with low-dose clonidine or beta-blocker based on the patients' symptoms.[21,33] Although a dexmedetomidine loading dose will decrease your time to sedation onset, it is often associated with hemodynamic instability and, therefore, should be not be used in hemodynamically unstable patients. Dexmedetomidine would not be a practical choice for patients requiring deep sedation.[23]

Propofol

Propofol is an IV sedative-hypnotic used commonly for anesthesia and ICU sedation. Because of its quick onset and short half-life, it is indicated for induction and maintenance of anesthesia and sedation. It is thought that propofol's sedative effects are mostly attributed to its positive modulation of the inhibitory function of the neurotransmitter γ-aminobutyric acid (GABA) on the $GABA_A$ receptor. Benefits of propofol include hypnotic, anxiolytic, amnestic, antiemetic, and anticonvulsant properties. Acutely, propofol can cause a dose-dependent respiratory depression and hypotension, especially when used with opioid medications. These effects are also more pronounced in patients already experiencing respiratory or cardiovascular insufficiency. With extended use, propofol can lead to hypertriglyceridemia and acute pancreatitis secondary to its lipid emulsion vehicle. The 10% lipid emulsion vehicle also contains egg lecithin and soybean oil; therefore, propofol should be avoided in patients with egg or soy allergies.[23] Propofol infusion syndrome is a rare and potentially lethal condition that has been associated with the administration of propofol infusions. The condition is most commonly characterized by cardiac failure, rhabdomyolysis, severe metabolic acidosis, renal failure, hyperkalemia, lipemia, hepatomegaly, or coved ST segment elevation. Patients at the highest risk are those receiving prolonged high doses of propofol (>83 mcg/kg/min for >48 hours).[22] Use of analgosedation may decrease this risk by allowing the practitioner to use lower doses of propofol.[34]

Benzodiazepines

Benzodiazepines activate the $GABA_A$ receptors in the brain. Similar to propofol, they have anxiolytic, amnestic, sedating, hypnotic, and anticonvulsant effects. Also similar to propofol, acutely, benzodiazepines cause respiratory depression and hypotension. These adverse effects are worsened when given concomitantly with opioids or in patients with baseline respiratory or cardiac insufficiency. Midazolam is typically preferred over lorazepam for short-term sedation (<48 hours) because of its short half-life when used for less than 48 hours and its lower potency. With prolonged use, however, midazolam and its active metabolites begin to accumulate; its use is associated with delayed awakening and longer ventilator times compared with lorazepam. The benzodiazepines are metabolized by the liver and cleared by the kidneys. Patients with renal or hepatic dysfunction and elderly patients will have prolonged effects. Propylene glycol is a common diluent in lorazepam solution. Propylene glycol toxicity can occur with cumulative dosages of 1 mg/kg/d of IV lorazepam. Toxicity manifests as a metabolic acidosis and acute kidney injury. It is important to monitor patients' serum osmol gap. An osmol gap greater than 10 to 12 mOsm/L would indicate possible propylene glycol toxicity.[23,24]

Analgosedation

Analgosedation, also known as analgesia-first sedation, is a validated sedative approach that uses opiates and pain management for patients' agitation instead of hypnotic sedatives. Analgosedation not only ensures that patients' pain is adequately treated but most of the opioids produce a sedative effect at higher doses. Currently recommended opioids for analgosedation are remifentanil and fentanyl as they can be easily titrated and have less concern of accumulation in organ failure. Morphine has been studied as well but is considered a second-line agent. The clinician should consider the addition of dexmedetomidine or propofol for rescue therapy for uncontrolled agitation.[24,34]

SEDATIVES AND ICU DELIRIUM

It is important to remember that sedatives are commonly associated with patients developing ICU delirium, which can have detrimental effects, including higher risk of mortality. Although data are conflicting for most drugs and their association with ICU delirium, most studies show that benzodiazepine use increases the risk of ICU patients transitioning to delirium. Furthermore, dexmedetomidine infusions have a lower association to the development of delirium when compared with benzodiazepines. As there are no currently recommended pharmacologic therapies for the treatment of ICU delirium, it is reasonable to minimize risk factors for delirium, which would include minimizing the use of benzodiazepines.[23,31,32,35]

SUMMARY

Pain and agitation may be difficult to assess in a critically ill patient. Pain is best assessed by self-reporting pain scales; but in patients who are unable to communicate, behavioral pain scales seem to have benefit. Patients' sedation level should be assessed each shift and preferably by a validated ICU tool, such as the RASS or SAS scale. Pain is most appropriately treated with the use of opiates, and careful consideration should be given to the pharmacokinetic and pharmacodynamic properties of various analgesics to determine the optimal agent for each individual patient. Sedation levels should preferably remain light or with the use of a daily awakening trial. Preferred treatment of agitation is analgosedation with the addition of nonbenzodiazepine sedatives if necessary. There are risks associated with each agent used in the treatment of pain and agitation, and it is important to monitor patients for effectiveness, signs of toxicity, and adverse drug reactions.

REFERENCES

1. Barr J, Files LF, Puntillo K, et al. Clinical practice guidelines for management of pain, agitation, and delirium in adult patients in the intensive care unit. Crit Care Med 2013;41(1):263–306.
2. Shapiro BA, Warren J, Egol AB, et al. Practice parameters for intravenous analgesia and sedation for adult patients in the intensive care unit: an executive summary. Society of Critical Care Medicine. Crit Care Med 1995;23(9):1596–600.
3. Jacobi J, Fraser GL, Coursin DB, et al, Task Force of the American College of Critical Care Medicine (ACCM) of the Society of Critical Care Medicine (SCCM), American Society of Health-System Pharmacists (ASHP), American College of Chest Physicians. Clinical practice guidelines for the sustained use of sedatives and analgesics in the critically ill adult. Crit Care Med 2002;30: 119–41.
4. Rotondi AJ, Chelluri L, Sirio C, et al. Patients' recollections of stressful experiences while receiving prolonged mechanical ventilation in an intensive care unit. Crit Care Med 2002;30:746–52.

5. Schelling G, Richter M, Roozendaal B, et al. Exposure to high stress in the intensive care unit may have negative effects on health-related quality-of-life outcomes after cardiac surgery. Crit Care Med 2003;31:1971–80.

6. Chanques G, Sebbane M, Barbotte E, et al. A prospective study of pain at rest: incidence and characteristics of an unrecognized symptom in surgical and trauma versus medical intensive care unit patients. Anesthesiology 2007;107:858–60.

7. Payen JF, Chanques G, Mantz J, et al. Current practices in sedation and analgesia for mechanically ventilated critically ill patients: a prospective multicenter patient-based study. Anesthesiology 2007;106:687–95 [quiz: 891].

8. Aïssaoui Y, Zeggwagh AA, Zekraoui A, et al. Validation of a behavioral pain scale in critically ill, sedated, and mechanically ventilated patients. Anesth Analg 2005; 101:1470–6.

9. Gélinas C, Johnston C. Pain assessment in the critically ill ventilated adult: validation of the critical-care pain observation tool and physiologic indicators. Clin J Pain 2007;23:497–505.

10. Payen JF, Bru O, Bosson JL, et al. Assessing pain in critically ill sedated patients by using a behavioral pain scale. Crit Care Med 2001;29:2258–63.

11. Gélinas C, Arbour C. Behavioral and physiologic indicators during a nociceptive procedure in conscious and unconscious mechanically ventilated adults: similar or different? J Crit Care 2009;24:628.e7–17.

12. Chanques G, Jaber S, Barbotte E, et al. Impact of systematic evaluation of pain and agitation in an intensive care unit. Crit Care Med 2006;34:1691–9.

13. Arbour C, Gélinas C, Michaud C. Impact of the implementation of the critical care pain observation tool (CPOT) on pain management and clinical outcomes in mechanically ventilated trauma intensive care unit patients: a pilot study. J Trauma Nurs 2011;18:52–60.

14. Gélinas C, Fillion L, Puntillo KA, et al. Validation of the critical care pain observation tool in adult patients. Am J Crit Care 2006;15:420–7.

15. Young J, Siffleet J, Nikoletti S, et al. Use of a behavioral pain scale to assess pain in ventilated, unconscious and/or sedated patients. Intensive Crit Care Nurs 2006;22:32–9.

16. Carrer S, Bocchi A, Candini M, et al. Short term analgesia based sedation in the intensive care unit: morphine vs remifentanil + morphine. Minerva Anestesiol 2007;73:327–32.

17. Maddali MM, Kurian E, Fahr J. Extubation time, hemodynamic stability, and postoperative pain control in patients undergoing coronary artery bypass surgery: an evaluation of fentanyl, remifentanil, and nonsteroidal antiinflammatory drugs with propofol for perioperative and postoperative management. J Clin Anesth 2006; 18:605–10.

18. Frakes MA, Lord WR, Kociszewski C, et al. Efficacy of fentanyl analgesia for trauma in critical care transport. Am J Emerg Med 2006;24:286–9.

19. Devlin JW, Roberts RJ. Pharmacology of commonly used analgesics and sedatives in the ICU: benzodiazepines, propofol, and opioids. Crit Care Clin 2009; 25:431–49, vii.

20. Muellejans B, López A, Cross MH, et al. Remifentanil versus fentanyl for analgesia based sedation to provide patient comfort in the intensive care unit: a randomized, double-blind controlled trial [ISRCTN42955713]. Crit Care 2004;8:R1–11.

21. Precedex (dexmedetomidine hydrochloride) [package insert]. Lake Forest, IL: Hospira; 2014.

22. Diprivan (propofol) [package insert]. Lake Zurich, IL: Fresenius Kabi USA, LLC; 2014.

23. Hypnovel (midazolam) [package insert]. Australia: Roche; 2015.

24. Ativan (lorazepam) [package insert]. Eatontown, NJ: West-Ward Pharmaceuticals; 2011.

25. Chou R, Cruciani RA, Fiellin DA, et al. Methadone safety: a clinical practice guideline from the American Pain Society and College on problems of drug dependence, in collaboration with the Heart Rhythm Society. J Pain 2014;15: 321–9.

26. Guillou N, Tanguy M, Seguin P, et al. The effects of small dose ketamine on morphine consumption in surgical intensive care unit patients after major abdominal surgery. Anesth Analg 2003;97:843–7.

27. Pandey CK, Bose N, Garg G, et al. Gabapentin for the treatment of pain in Guillainbarré syndrome: a double-blinded, placebo-controlled, crossover study. Anesth Analg 2002;95:1719–23.

28. Pandey CK, Raza M, Tripathi M, et al. The comparative evaluation of gabapentin and carbamazepine for pain management in GuillainBarré syndrome patients in the intensive care unit. Anesth Analg 2005;101:220–5.

29. Girard TD, Kress JP, Fuchs BD, et al. Efficacy and safety of a paired sedation and ventilator weaning protocol for mechanically ventilated patients in the intensive care (awakening and breathing controlled trial): a randomized controlled trial. Lancet 2008;371:126–34.

30. Fraser GL, Devlin JW, Worby CP, et al. Benzodiazepine versus nonbenzodiazepine-based sedation for mechanically ventilated, critically ill adults: a systematic review and meta-analysis of randomized trials. Crit Care Med 2013;41(9 Suppl 1):S30–8.

31. Riker RR, Shehabi Y, Bokesch PM, et al. Dexmedetomidine vs midazolam for sedation of critically ill patients: a randomized trial. JAMA 2009;301(5):489–99.

32. Pandharipande PP, Pun BT, Herr DL, et al. Effect of sedation with dexmedetomidine vs lorazepam on acute brain dysfunction in mechanically ventilated patients: the MENDS randomized controlled trial. JAMA 2007;298(22):2644–53.

33. Weber MA. Discontinuation syndrome following cessation of treatment with clonidine and other antihypertensive agents. J Cardiovasc Pharmacol 1980;2(Suppl 1):S73–89.

34. Devabhakthuni S, Armahizer MJ, Dasta JF, et al. Analgosedation: a paradigm shift in intensive care unit sedation practice. Ann Pharmacother 2012;46(4): 530–40.

35. Pandharipande PP, Girard TD, Jackson JC, et al. Long-term cognitive impairment after critical illness. N Engl J Med 2013;369(14):1306–16.

Immunosuppressive Therapy in Transplantation

Terri L. Allison, DNP, ACNP-BC, FAANP

KEYWORDS

- Immunosuppression • Immunosuppressive medications • Transplantation
- Hematopoietic stem cell transplantation

KEY POINTS

- Organ and hematopoietic stem cell transplants are lifesaving treatment options for patients with end-stage organ failure or life-threatening blood or bone marrow disorders.
- Immunosuppressive medications are given to modulate the transplant recipient's immune response to the donor organ or tissue, including induction, maintenance, and rescue therapy.
- Patient management and consideration of the complex immunosuppressive regimen are essential for long-term patient and graft survival and enhanced patient outcomes.
- Health care providers must understand the implications of immunosuppressive medications, including dosing strategies; the monitoring required; and associated side effects, complications, adverse events, and concomitant medication interactions.

INTRODUCTION

Organ transplant can be a lifesaving treatment option for patients with end-stage organ failure. Stem cell transplant is a treatment option for those with blood cancer, bone marrow failure, or other immune system or genetic disorders.[1] Because transplantation involves implanting recipients with an organ or tissue (graft) from a donor with different immune proteins, transplantation presents many immunologic challenges. A consequence of transplanting divergent donor immune proteins and the leading cause of graft failure is rejection among organ transplant recipients and graft-versus-host disease (GVHD) among hematopoietic stem cell transplant (HSCT) recipients.[2,3] Rejection and GVHD are complex immune responses mediated by mononuclear cells, such as macrophages and dendritic cells; B and T lymphocytes; cytokines, interleukin-2 (IL-2), in particular with organ transplantation; multiple inflammatory mediators with GVHD; and complement.[4] Patient survival, and functioning of

Disclosures: None.

Doctor of Nursing Practice Program, Vanderbilt University School of Nursing, 461 21st Avenue, South 603D Godchaux Hall, Nashville, TN 37240, USA

E-mail address: terri.allison@vanderbilt.edu

Nurs Clin N Am 51 (2016) 107–120
http://dx.doi.org/10.1016/j.cnur.2015.10.008
0029-6465/16/$ – see front matter © 2016 Elsevier Inc. All rights reserved.

the transplanted organ or stem cells, depend on modulation of the immune system to prevent graft failure. A complex medication regimen, not commonly seen in routine patient care, is used to suppress the recipient's immune response to the transplanted tissue. Health care providers involved in the care of patients undergoing transplants must understand the use of these medications and dosing strategies, as well as side effects and the associated complications. In addition, most immunosuppressants are metabolized via the cytochrome P (CYP) 450 enzyme pathway and are subject to significant food and drug interactions, contributing the complexity of management of this patient population.

Transplant medication regimens are given throughout different periods during and after transplant and serve several purposes. Induction therapy is immunosuppression administered just before, during, and/or immediately after the transplant to prevent organ rejection.[5] An induction agent may also be administered in the immediate postoperative period to avoid administration of nephrotoxic immunosuppressants to preserve kidney function or to allow steroid-free transplant.[6] Maintenance immunosuppression usually comprises 3 medications taken by the recipient in doses to prevent rejection or GVHD while allowing the immune system to maintain enough function to fight infection. Over time, in some types of transplants, the initial 3 medications may be reduced to 2 or even 1 medication, or a medication selected for maintenance is replaced by another because of an untoward side effect, complication, or rejection episode. Rescue therapy involves administration of additional immunosuppressants to treat a rejection episode or worsening GVHD.[7] When rejection or GVHD occurs, doses of the recipient's maintenance medications may be augmented or a maintenance drug may be replaced with another to enhance the effectiveness of the maintenance regimen in conjunction with the rescue therapy.

Immunosuppression is fraught with side effects, complications, and adverse events.[8] Although drug-free tolerance of the transplant is the optimal goal,[9] no effective methods have been developed to allow immunosuppressant-free transplant. Careful management of the patient and consideration of the individualized immunosuppressive regimen are essential for long-term patient and graft survival and enhanced patient outcomes.[8] Many immunosuppressive agents used in organ and hematopoietic stem cell (HSC) transplantation do not have approved indications for all types of transplants performed and are thus used off-label to prevent rejection or GVHD.

Pharmacologic trials often test new drugs in kidney or liver transplant recipients because of the particular characteristics associated with these organs. Kidney transplant is considered a life-enhancing treatment; therefore, if renal graft failure occurs, patients have another renal replacement option with dialysis. The liver is an immunologically privileged organ,[10] thus the threshold for rejection is higher and the liver's regenerative capabilities result in less injury if rejection does occur.[11] However, because the mechanisms of immunologic graft failure and GVHD are similar, the utility of these immunosuppressant medications generalizes across all types of transplants.[12]

INDUCTION THERAPY

Induction therapy provides intense, short-term immunosuppression during the perioperative transplant period to overlap with administration of maintenance therapy to prevent rejection and improve outcomes.[4,7,13–15] Induction therapy is routine in most kidney transplants, is institution specific with other organs, and has been shown to reduce acute rejection rates and graft survival.[4,7,16] An analysis of data from the United

Network for Organ Sharing Registry showed that induction therapy improved graft and patient outcomes for most organ transplants.[15,17] Use of an induction agent also permits postponement of calcineurin inhibitor (CNI) administration to prevent early onset nephrotoxicity or provides potent immunosuppression in the setting of steroid-free transplantation.[7,18] Induction agents available are either monoclonal or polyclonal antibodies that deplete or prevent clonal expansion of T lymphocytes that mediate transplant rejection and GVHD.[6,7] Equine antithymocyte globulin (E-ATG) and rabbit antithymocyte globulin (R-ATG) are polyclonal antibodies; basiliximab (Simulect) and alemtuzumab (Campath) are monoclonal antibodies (**Table 1**). R-ATG is more effective in preventing acute rejection compared with E-ATG and is the preferred polyclonal agent that depletes the T lymphocytes from circulation.[4,7,16] R-ATG requires intravenous dosing at 1 to 4 mg/kg/d for 3 to 10 days posttransplant.[19] The most problematic

Table 1
Induction agents

Medication, Generic (Brand Name)	Administration	Management
Antithymocyte globulin • R-ATG (thymoglobulin) • E-ATG (Atgam)	E-ATG: 10–20 mg/kg/d IV over 6–8 h via central line R-ATG: 1.25–1.5 mg/kg/d IV over 6–8 h first dose, 4–6 h subsequent doses; central line preferred	• Premedicate: methylprednisolone, diphenhydramine, acetaminophen • Skin test with E-ATG, none with R-ATG • Side effects: anaphylaxis, fever, chills, flulike symptoms, thrombocytopenia, infection • Monitoring: CBC, B-cell and T-cell subsets, antiequine or rabbit polyclonal IgG antibody to test for sensitization • Duration of therapy 3–10 d for induction, 7–14 d if treating acute rejection or GVHD
Basiliximab (Simulect)	20 mg IV over 15 min on days 0 and 4 via peripheral or central line	Side effects: hypotension, hypersensitivity reaction, tachycardia, bronchospasm, pulmonary edema, infection
Alemtuzumab (Campath)	30 mg IV over 2 h × 1 dose for induction 10 mg IV daily × 5 d, then weekly for GVHD	• Premedicate: methylprednisolone, diphenhydramine, acetaminophen • Side effects: anaphylaxis, pancytopenia, infusion site reactions, fever, chills, flulike symptoms, infection • Monitoring: CBC, absolute lymphocyte count, antimurine monoclonal antibody to test for sensitization • Duration of therapy longer if treating GVHD

Abbreviations: CBC, complete blood count; IgG, immunoglobulin G; IV, intravenous.

Data from Chaballa M, Filicko-O'Hara J, Holt D, et al. Transplant medicine. In: Waldman SA, editor. Pharmacology and therapeutics: principles to practice. Philadelphia: Saunders; 2009. p. 1269–94; and Vo AA, Chaux GE, Falk JA. Transplant pharmacology. In: Lewis ML, editor. Medical management of the thoracic surgery patient. Philadelphia: Saunders; 2010. p. 352–6.

adverse effect of the polyclonal antibodies is cytokine release creating flulike symptoms of fever, chills, headache, nausea, diarrhea, and malaise, and in rare cases anaphylaxis.[7,19,20] Patients are premedicated with diphenhydramine and acetaminophen to ameliorate symptoms caused by cytokine release.[7]

Alemtuzumab is a recombinant DNA-derived monoclonal antibody with no clear consensus about appropriate dosing, and seems to be most effective in low-immunologic-risk recipients. Alemtuzumab has shown poorer outcomes compared with R-ATG; its current use as an induction agent is therefore limited.[7,16] Basiliximab is the only antibody approved by the US Food and Drug Administration (FDA) for induction therapy; all other induction agents are used off-label. Basiliximab requires intravenous administration in a 2-dose regimen of 20 mg 2 hours before transplant and repeated on postoperative day 4.[6,7,20] The immunologic effects of basiliximab persist 5 to 8 weeks posttransplant, resulting in profound immunosuppression. The drug is well tolerated with few adverse effects; however, basiliximab has a boxed warning for hypersensitivity reactions, although they rarely occur.[7]

Induction therapy is controversial. Even though induction therapy provides clear improvement in patient and graft outcomes, infection and malignancy, particularly cytomegalovirus and lymphoma respectively, remain major concerns following administration of induction therapy.[6,13,14,19,21] Basiliximab seems to result in fewer infections compared with other agents.[5] Further data are needed to determine whether basiliximab is superior to R-ATG in the reduced incidence of neoplasm. More research is needed to determine long-term outcomes of induction therapy, particularly involving the newer agents, to determine incidence of infection and malignancy and the relationship to patient and graft survival.

Administration of a monoclonal or polyclonal antibody is effective in the prevention of GVHD; however, the therapy is problematic in that the drug can delay immune reconstitution, making HSCT recipients more susceptible to life-threatening infection, graft failure, and recurrence of disease.[21] R-ATG is recommended for prevention of chronic GVHD and has been shown to improve quality of life in HSCT recipients who receive cells from a nonrelated donor.[22] Effectiveness in the prevention and treatment of GVHD with R-ATG in patients receiving related donor HSCT is unknown.

MAINTENANCE IMMUNOSUPPRESSIVE THERAPY

Maintenance immunosuppression uses multiple medications to target different regions of the immune response to prevent rejection or GVHD.[7,18] Historically in organ transplantation, immunosuppression comprised azathioprine and corticosteroids.[7] A cytotoxic agent or total body irradiation to suppress the bone marrow production of lymphocytes was also used as a method of rejection prophylaxis.[2] These regimens were problematic in that the medications and irradiation were nonspecific and inadequate to achieve the level of immunosuppression necessary to prevent rejection while avoiding oversuppression of the immune system. Maintenance immunosuppressive medications must be carefully selected and dosages titrated to prevent rejection while minimizing complications and toxicities.[7,23] Transplant immunosuppression entered a new era with improved patient and graft survival in the early 1980s with the advent of cyclosporine (CsA), a CNI.[4] At present, maintenance immunosuppression most often comprises a 3-drug regimen including a CNI, an antiproliferative agent, and corticosteroids.[2,23] A mammalian target of rapamycin (mTOR) inhibitor may replace the CNI or be added to the 3-drug regimen for patients who experience significant adverse effects from the CNI or have recurrent rejection epidsodes.[7] Doses of immunosuppressants are highest in the first months following the transplant and gradually tapered to maintenance doses over the first year to minimize toxicity.[23] Immunosuppression is lifelong in organ transplant recipients, although the 3-drug regimen may be reduced to 2 medications, or in rare instances to 1, whereas HSCT recipients are often able to withdraw from immunosuppression entirely because most patients achieve a state of tolerance between recipient tissues and donor immune responses.[3,19]

Generic forms are available for several immunosuppressant agents used in organ and HSC transplantation; however, clinical trial data regarding bioequivalence and efficacy of these medications are lacking.[24] Further complicating medication management is that multiple generic compounds are available and different generic formulations may be dispensed at the pharmacy with subsequent refills.[25] Available data to date have not shown adverse patient outcomes when using generic preparations, but the narrow therapeutic index associated with immunosuppression necessitates careful monitoring of therapeutic drug levels, patient tolerance, and graft function to minimize complications when the recipient changes from brand name formulations to generic or with changes in the generic drug manufacturer of the prescribed medications.[25,26] Maintenance immunosuppressive agents, doses, adverse effects, and particular patient management concerns are described in **Table 2**.

Calcineurin Inhibitors

CsA and tacrolimus (TAC) are CNIs that block IL-2 and T lymphocytes; the primary mediators of graft rejection and GVHD.[4] The CNIs are the mainstay for prevention of rejection and GVHD.[6,7,27] The original oil-based formulation of CsA, known as Sandimmune, has unpredictable absorption and is infrequently used.[6,7] CsA microemulsion (CsA-modified), available by the brand names of Neoral and Gengraf as well as in generic form, is the preferred formulation because of greater bioavailability and predictable absorption.[6] CsA microemulsion is available in oral solution and capsule. Sandimmune is the only CsA formulation available for intravenous administration via continuous infusion if oral administration is contraindicated.[7] CsA and CsA-modified are not bioequivalent and thus are not interchangeable. Prescribers must ensure that the appropriate preparation, and preferably a consistent name brand or generic formulation, is dispensed to patients.[28]

CsA dosing is 5 to 10 mg/kg administered in divided doses every 12 hours. Regular and evenly spaced timing of medication administration is important to maintaining a consistent therapeutic blood level. Dosing adjustments are made based on therapeutic trough drug levels, the goal of which is determined by the organ or tissue involved, time since transplant, and institution-specific and patient-specific therapeutic drug level targets.[7] Goal therapeutic CsA levels are highest in the weeks following transplant. If the recipient remains rejection free, the dose is reduced to achieve a lower therapeutic drug level to minimize drug toxicity.

TAC, also known by the chemical name FK-506, is a macrolide antibiotic with properties similar to CsA. Brand name (Prograf) and generic formulations are available and administered in 2 divided doses every 12 hours to achieve the desired therapeutic drug level. TAC is available in capsule and intravenous form; however, TAC is seldom given parenterally because of toxicity and the potential for anaphylaxis.[7] As with CsA, goal therapeutic levels are highest in the early weeks posttransplant and then reduced over time because of significant toxic effects of the agent.

Although the development of CNIs was the turning point in successful transplantation and remains the mainstay of immunosuppression, they have an extensive adverse effect profile. Problems associated with CNIs are similar between CsA and TAC; the most common include nephrotoxicity; hypertension; neurotoxicity manifesting as headache, hand tremors, or seizure; hyperlipidemia; hyperuricemia; hyperkalemia;

Table 2
Maintenance immunosuppression

Medication (Brand Name)	Common Dosage	Adverse Effects	Management
• CsA (Sandimmune) • CsA-modified (Neoral, Gengraf, multiple generics)	Oral: 5–10 mg/kg/d divided every 12 h, capsules or suspension IV: one-third of oral dose continuous infusion every 12 h	Hypertension, neurotoxicity, nephrotoxicity, gingival hyperplasia, hirsutism, hyperlipidemia, glucose intolerance, hypomagnesemia	• CsA and CsA-modified not bioequivalent • TDM: 12 h trough 3 d after any change or when clinically indicated • BMP for creatinine, glucose, magnesium
TAC, FK-506 (Prograf, generics)	Oral: 0.05–0.2 mg/kg/d divided every 12 h IV: one-third of oral dose continuous infusion every 12 h	Hypertension, neurotoxicity, nephrotoxicity, alopecia, glucose intolerance, hypomagnesemia, hyperkalemia	• IV form may cause anaphylaxis; avoid if possible • TDM: 12 h trough 3 d after any change or when clinically indicated • BMP: less hyperlipidemia, hypertension; more glucose intolerance compared with CsA
AZA (Imuran, generic)	Oral: 1–3 mg/kg/d IV: 1:1 conversion	Pancytopenia, nausea, vomiting, diarrhea, pancreatitis, liver toxicity, alopecia	• CBC with platelets • Discontinue if WBC <3000 cells/mm^3 • Hepatic function tests
MMF (CellCept, generic)	Oral: 1–1.5 g every 12 h IV: 1 g every 12 h	GI distress, cytopenias	• TDM available but not routinely done • CBC
MPS (Myfortic)	Oral: 360–720 g every 12 h No IV formulation	Gastrointestinal distress, cytopenias	• TDM available but not routinely done • CBC
Sirolimus (Rapamune, generic tablets)	Oral loading dose: 3–6 mg, up to 15 mg for high risk, then 1–3 mg daily; 5 mg high risk; solution or tablets No IV formulation	Thrombocytopenia, hyperlipidemia, especially triglycerides, impaired wound healing, pneumonitis, GI distress, aphthous ulcers	• Higher dose for high-risk patients • TDM 12-h trough 5–7 d after initiation • Administer 4 h after CsA • CBC, lipid levels

Drug	Dosing	Adverse effects	Monitoring/Comments
Everolimus (Zortress)	Oral: 0.75–1 mg every 12 h, tablets or oral suspension (formulations not interchangeable) No IV formulation	Pneumonitis, hepatic toxicity, infection, hypertension, peripheral edema, GI distress, hyperlipidemia, angioedema, cytopenias, graft thrombosis, malignancy, mucositis/stomatitis, nephrotoxicity, delayed wound healing	• TDM at intervals of 4–5 d as needed • Administer at same time as TAC or CsA • Liver: in combination with reduced-dose TAC and steroids • Kidney: in combination with basiliximab induction, dose-adjusted CsA and steroids • Contraindicated in heart transplant
Corticosteroids • Methylprednisolone (Solu-Medrol) • Prednisone (Deltasone, Medrol)	Methylprednisolone, IV: • Initial: 250–1000 mg daily × 1–3 d • Rejection: 5–10 mg/kg daily × 3 Prednisone, oral: • Maintenance: dependent on center protocol; tapered to 2.5–5 mg once daily or discontinued • Rejection: bump and taper, dosing center dependent	Hypertension, fluid retention, increased appetite, weight gain, cushingoid features, avascular necrosis of bone, osteoporosis, hyperglycemia, steroid-induced diabetes, proximal myopathy, mood disturbance, psychosis, impaired wound healing, peptic ulcer, GI bleeding, adrenal insufficiency, cataracts, glaucoma, infection	• Clinical and laboratory monitoring for adverse reactions • CBC, lipid panel, electrolytes, glucose • Blood pressure, weight, temperature • Increased WBC expected at initiation because of demarginalization

Abbreviations: AZA, azathioprine; BMP, basic metabolic panel; GI, gastrointestinal; MMF, mycophenolate mofetil; MPS, mycophenolate sodium; TDM, therapeutic drug monitoring; WBC, white blood cell count.

Data from Chaballa M, Filicko-O'Hara J, Holt D, et al. Transplant medicine. In: Waldman SA, editor. Pharmacology and therapeutics: principles to practice. Philadelphia: Saunders; 2009. p. 1269–94; and Vo AA, Chaux GE, Falk JA. Transplant pharmacology. In: Lewis ML, editor. Medical management of the thoracic surgery patient. Philadelphia: Saunders; 2010. p. 352–6.

hypomagnesemia; and hyperglycemia.[4,7,19] CsA causes gingival hyperplasia and hirsutism, whereas TAC causes alopecia.[6] In addition, TAC has been shown to produce greater gastrointestinal distress and glucose intolerance, with fewer implications for hyperlipidemia and hypertension.[4,7] TAC has become the CNI of choice in many transplant centers because of demonstrated decrease in rejection episodes compared with CsA.[4,13,29]

CsA and TAC are metabolized via the CYP450 3A4 enzymes and therapeutic drug levels can be subject to variability caused by drug or food interactions metabolized via the same enzyme pathway[6,30] (**Table 3**). Side effects caused by CNI administration are numerous and patients often require frequent monitoring of therapeutic drug levels, attention to concomitant medication administration and interaction with certain foods and herbal supplements, as well as implementation of lifestyle adjustments to minimize adverse effects.

Antiproliferative Agents

Azathioprine, mycophenolate mofetil (MMF), and mycophenolate sodium are antimetabolites that interrupt the DNA synthesis phase of lymphocyte proliferation.[6] Azathioprine was one of the first drugs approved for use in transplantation and was the hallmark of immunosuppression until the development of CsA; however, the drug has been used much less frequently since the more specific inhibitor, MMF, became available.[7]

Azathioprine is a nonspecific antimetabolite causing myelosuppression that results in reduction of all hematopoietic cell lines. Anemia, leukocytopenia, and thrombocytopenia are common.[20] Azathioprine is known to cause alopecia, gastrointestinal distress, pancreatitis, and hepatotoxicity, and is more frequently implicated in the increased incidence of skin cancer posttransplant.[7,31] Dosing is 3 to 5 mg/kg given once daily, usually at bedtime; intravenous and oral forms are available. A complete blood count should be monitored for excessive pancytopenia at least every 3 months in stable transplant recipients, and more frequently initially after transplant. The most

Table 3		
Food and drug interactions with immunosuppression: CsA, TAC, sirolimus		
Substrates[a]	**Inducers[b]**	**Inhibitors[c]**
Amiodarone	Phenobarbital, phenytoin,	Clarithromycin, azithromycin,
Statins	carbamazepine	erythromycin
Dapsone	Rifampin	Itraconazole, ketoconazole, fluconazole,
Amlodipine, felodipine	Nafcillin	miconazole, voriconazole
Clonazepam, sertraline,	Orlistat	Diltiazem, verapamil
venlafaxine	St John's wort	Saquinavir, indinavir, nelfinavir, ritonavir
Warfarin		Cimetidine
Zolpidem		Ciprofloxacin
Benzodiazepines		Fluvoxamine
Omeprazole		Grapefruit juice

[a] Substrates compete for metabolism or drug transport; increased concentration of both drugs.
[b] Inducers enhanced drug metabolism/drug transport decreasing concentration of CsA, TAC, or sirolimus.
[c] Inhibitors decrease drug metabolism/drug transport increasing concentration of CsA, TAC, or sirolimus.
From Gabardi S, Tichy EM. Overview of immunosuppressive therapies in renal transplantation. In: Chadraker A, Sayegh MH, Singh AJ, editors. Core concepts in renal transplantation. New York: Springer; 2012. p. 121; with permission.

significant drug interaction is concomitant administration of allopurinol. If both medications are necessary, the azathioprine dose must be reduced by one-third to one-quarter to avoid severe myelosuppression.[6]

MMF (CellCept) and mycophenolate sodium (Myfortic) are prodrugs that are metabolized to the active form of mycophenolate acid (MPA), which inhibits lymphocytes.[6,7] MMF is superior to azathioprine and is the preferred antiproliferative routinely used in transplantation because of its increased efficacy in preventing rejection compared with azathioprine, ease of use, and improved side effect profile.[4,6,7] MMF in combination with a CNI shows synergistic effects in prevention of GVHD.[21] The drug comes in both brand name and generic oral capsule, and suspension and intravenous forms. Mycophenolate sodium is an enteric form of the MPA prodrug, and may be better tolerated by patients experiencing gastrointestinal distress with MMF.[6] MMF and mycophenolate sodium are not interchangeable because of differences in absorption and dosing. The dose of MMF is 2 to 3 g administered in divided doses every 12 hours.[7] Mycophenolate sodium dosing is 360 to 720 mg every 12 hours. Therapeutic drug monitoring is available for MMF but is not routinely performed because clinical utility is uncertain.[19] Major side effects of the MPA agents include gastrointestinal distress and myelosuppression.[7,20] Higher doses (>1 g) of MMF are more likely to cause significant gastrointestinal side effects; reduction in dose often resolves symptoms.[20]

Mammalian Target of Rapamycin Inhibitors

mTOR inhibitors, sirolimus (Rapamycin) and everolimus (Zortress), hinder lymphocyte activation and proliferation by blocking the response to cytokine stimulation.[6,7] Both agents are available commercially in oral form and are metabolized via the CYP450 3A4 system.[6,7] Sirolimus is indicated for high-immunologic-risk transplant recipients; everolimus is indicated for prevention of rejection in low-risk to moderate-risk recipients and given in conjunction with induction therapy, reduced-dose CsA, and corticosteroids.[7] Sirolimus may also be started in patients who do not tolerate a CNI or develop CNI nephrotoxicity.[6] Sirolimus is begun with a loading dose of 3 to 6 mg, followed by once-daily maintenance administration of 1 to 3 mg separated by 4 hours from administration of a CNI; the sirolimus dose must be reduced with hepatic impairment. Therapeutic drug monitoring can facilitate dosing and desired drug levels are determined by the recipient's immunologic risk. Initiation of an mTOR inhibitor is deferred for at least 30 days after transplant to avoid wound dehiscence and impaired wound healing.[32–35] If possible, sirolimus or everolimus should be discontinued 1 week before elective surgery and the agent resumed 10 to 15 days after surgery.[34] Other significant adverse events associated with mTOR inhibitors include hyperlipidemia, cytopenias, proteinuria, hypertension, and aphthous ulcers.[19,34] With concomitant use of sirolimus and CsA or TAC, the CNI dose must be reduced to avoid significant renal impairment.[6]

Because of concern for nephrotoxicity with long-term CNI administration, particularly in kidney transplantation, clinical trials were undertaken to determine the effectiveness of switching transplant recipients from CNI-based immunosuppression to an mTOR inhibitor. Study outcomes showed that changing patients with a functioning renal graft to sirolimus did not provide any long-term benefit.[36] Therefore, sirolimus does not provide greater renal protection compared with CNI with long-term use.

Corticosteroids

Steroids are nonspecific immunosuppressants that inhibit B and T lymphocytes and cytokines.[2,7,20] Methylprednisolone is administered intravenously in the intraoperative and immediate postoperative period, followed by oral prednisone. Dosing regimens vary based on organ transplant or HSCT, transplant center practices, and patient needs. Typically oral prednisone is given at 0.8 to 1 mg/kg per day in divided doses twice daily.[7] Oral corticosteroids are then tapered over subsequent weeks and months posttransplant. Depending on the type of transplant, steroids are stopped or reduced to a maintenance daily dose of 2.5 to 5 mg/d.[7] Adverse effects associated with chronic administration of steroids contribute to significant morbidity and reduced quality of life posttransplant, so doses are reduced as much and as quickly as possible. **Table 2** for descriptions of side effects associated with corticosteroids.

Biologic Agents

Belatacept (Nulojix) is a biologic agent in a new drug class approved in 2011 for prophylaxis of organ rejection in kidney transplant recipients.[7] The use of this agent is unique in that it can be used as maintenance immunosuppression to replace the CNI, in combination with basiliximab induction and standard immunosuppression with MMF and corticosteroids.[7,16,20] Belatacept has a complicated administration regimen and requires intravenous infusion over 30 minutes just before graft implantation, repeated on day 5, then every 2 weeks to week 12, then every 4 weeks beginning at week 16.[37,38] Even though belatacept has demonstrated effectiveness, the drug seems to result in higher incidence of lymphoma in transplant recipients who are Ebstein-Barr negative at the time of transplant,[39] and its use as routine immunosuppression is limited by its high cost.[16] As the newest immunosuppressant agent available, more data are needed to determine its place among the armamentarium of immunosuppressants.

RESCUE THERAPY

Rescue therapy is the administration of powerful immunosuppression to treat an acute organ rejection episode or the occurrence or exacerbation of GVHD in HSCT.[7,22] The first-line agent used to treat rejection or GVHD is corticosteroids.[7,18] With GVHD, oral prednisone is begun in divided doses at 2 mg/kg/d and then tapered as the GVHD resolves. Maintenance immunosuppression continues during the steroid taper and others are added if the GVHD persists or worsens during acute treatment.[19,22] Severe or unresponsive GVHD may be treated with a monoclonal or polyclonal antibody.

Biopsy-proven acute organ rejection is managed with high-dose oral prednisone or intravenous methylprednisolone.[7] The approach to treatment of acute rejection depends on the severity of the episode, the presence of organ dysfunction, and time since transplant. Methylprednisolone is dosed at 250 to 1000 mg intravenously daily, typically for 3 days. Rejection occurring early posttransplant, high-grade rejection, or rejection accompanied by organ dysfunction is typically treated with intravenous methylprednisolone. An alternative is increased oral prednisone given in high doses divided twice daily that is then tapered (bump and taper) over a period of days or weeks. Severe or high-grade, biopsy-proven rejection, with or without organ dysfunction, is treated with oral or intravenous corticosteroids and the polyclonal antibody, ATG. Dosing is consistent with the doses used when the drug is given as an induction agent. Alemtuzumab and basiliximab are not used for treatment of acute rejection.

FOOD AND DRUG INTERACTIONS

The CNIs and mTOR inhibitors are metabolized via the CYP450 3A4 enzyme pathway. Other medications that are substrates, inducers, or inhibitors of CYP450 3A4 can cause significant derangements in effectiveness or the side effect profile of immunosuppressants. Substrates compete with CNIs and mTOR inhibitors and potentially increase immunosuppressant concentrations by as much as 20%.[7] Medications that inhibit CYP 3A4 decrease drug metabolism, resulting in increased serum concentrations of CsA, TAC, and sirolimus, whereas 3A4 inducers increase drug metabolism and reduce therapeutic drug levels of these agents[7,30] (see **Table 3**). Concomitant administration of medications with similar adverse events to the CNIs and sirolimus can result in untoward additive effects.[7] For example, amphotericin B and the aminoglycosides are known to be nephrotoxic.[7] Use with CsA, TAC, or sirolimus can precipitate acute or chronic renal failure if not carefully monitored and doses reduced. Nonsteroidal antiinflammatory drugs can increase the risk of nephrotoxicity and hypertension in combination with CNIs.

Interactions affecting the mycophenolate preparations are primarily related to changes in gastric and intestinal absorption. Aluminum, magnesium, or calcium products, or any of the bile sequestrants, must be administered at least 2 hours before or 1 hour following the MPA drugs to avoid decreased effectiveness of immunosuppression.[7] Azathioprine is metabolized outside the CYP system but has significant interaction with allopurinol.[7] Combined use of azathioprine and allopurinol can cause severe myelosuppression. If allopurinol must be given, reduce the azathioprine dose by 75% and monitor the complete blood count.[20] A preferred alternative is to replace azathioprine with MMF before starting allopurinol to avoid this significant drug interaction.

Most immunosuppressants are labeled with a boxed warning from the FDA, which is the most serious type of warning mandated to alert providers about serious adverse reactions.[40] Boxed warnings appear with the prescribing information. Immunosuppressant medications used in transplantation should only be prescribed by providers familiar with the agents used, doses, side effects, and therapeutic monitoring required.

SUMMARY

Transplantation offers patients with end-stage organ failure or life-threatening blood or bone marrow disorders an opportunity for enhanced survival and quality of life. Survival of this patient population depends on alteration of the immune system with immunosuppression to mediate the body's response to the transplanted organ or tissue. Immunosuppression, although essential, is a complex and demanding medical regimen that requires providers to exercise vigilance to ensure appropriate medication dosing, monitoring for adverse events and complications, and awareness of a multitude of food and drug interactions. Current and future initiatives in transplantation will focus on modalities to achieve tolerance of the transplanted organ or tissue to improve long-term outcomes while minimizing toxicities associated with immunosuppression. Providers will need to remain appraised of implications of these new modalities as the art and science of transplantation evolve.

REFERENCES

1. Understanding transplantation as a treatment option. US Department of Health and Human Services Health Resources and Services Administration Web site. Available at: http://bloodcell.transplant.hrsa.gov/transplant/understanding_tx/index.html. Accessed September 1, 2015.
2. Mancini MC, Cush EM, Launius BK, et al. The management of immunosuppression: the art and the science. Crit Care Nurs Q 2004;27(1):61–4.
3. Socié G, Blazar B. Overview of immune biology of allogenic hematopoietic stem cell transplantation. In: Socié G, Blazar B, editors. Immune biology of allogeneic hematopoietic stem cell transplantation. Boston: Elsevier; 2013. p. 1–17. Available

at: http://www.sciencedirect.com.proxy.library.vanderbilt.edu/science/article/pii/B978012416004000001X. Accessed September 7, 2015.

4. Hricik D. Transplant immunology and immunosuppression: core curriculum 2015. Am J Kidney Dis 2015;65(6):956–66.

5. Liu Y, Zouh P, Han M, et al. Basiliximab or antithymocyte globulin for induction therapy in kidney transplantation: a meta-analysis. Transplant Proc 2010;42(5):1667–70.

6. Wojciechowski D, Veilette G, Vincenti F. Immunosuppression with the kidney as paradigm. In: Forsythe JLR, editor. Transplantation. 5th edition. Philadelphia: Elsevier; 2014. p. 67–88. Available at: https://www-clinicalkey-com.proxy.library.vanderbilt.edu/#!/browse/book/3-s2.0-C20110057216. Accessed September 1, 2015.

7. Gibardi S, Tichy EM. Overview of immunosuppressive therapies in renal transplantation. In: Chandrakar A, Sayegh MH, Singh AJ, editors. Core concepts in renal transplantation. New York: Springer; 2012. p. 97–127. Available at: http://link.springer.com.proxy.library.vanderbilt.edu/book/10.1007%2F978-1-4614-0008-0. Accessed September 1, 2015.

8. Eisen HJ. Immunosuppression-state-of-the-art: anything new in the pipeline? Curr Opin Organ Transplant 2014;19(5):500–7.

9. Flechner SM. Optimizing immunosuppression: who can do more with less? Transpl Int 2015. http://dx.doi.org/10.1111/tri.12676.

10. Sumpter T, Abe M, Tokita D, et al. Dendritic cells, the liver and transplantation. Hepatology 2007;46(6):2021–31.

11. Zhang Q, Rjalingam R, Cecka JM, et al. ABO, tissue typing, and crossmatch incompatibility. In: Busuttil RW, Klintmalm GBG, editors. Transplantation of the Liver. 3rd edition. Philadelphia: Saunders; 2015. p. 1245–56. Available at: https://www-clinicalkey-com.proxy.library.vanderbilt.edu/#!/browse/book/3-s2.0-B978072160118 2X50010. Accessed September 1, 2015.

12. Bennett WM. Off-label use of approved drugs: therapeutic opportunity and challenges. J Am Soc Nephrol 2004;15(3):830–1.

13. Aliabadi A, Cochrane AB, Zuckermann AO. Current strategies and future trends in immunosuppression after heart transplantation. Curr Opin Organ Transplant 2012;17(5):540–5.

14. Laftavi MR, Sharma R, Feng L, et al. Induction therapy in renal transplant recipients: a review. Immunol Invest 2014;43(8):790–806.

15. Whitson BA, Lehman A, Wehr A. To induce or not to induce: a 21st century evaluation of lung transplant immunosuppression's effect on survival. Clin Transplant 2014;28(4):450–61.

16. Wohlfahrtova M, Viklicky O. Recent trials in immunosuppression and their consequences for current therapy. Curr Opin Organ Transplant 2014;19(4):387–94.

17. Cai J, Terasaki PI. Induction immunosuppression improves long-term graft and patient outcome in organ transplantation: an analysis of United Network for Organ Sharing registry data. Transplantation 2010;90(12):1511–5.

18. Wiesner RH, Fung JL. Present state of immunosuppressive therapy in liver transplant recipients. Liver Transplant 2011;17(S3):S1–9.

19. Chaballa M, Filicko-O'Hara J, Holt D, et al. Transplant medicine. In: Waldman SA, editor. Pharmacology and therapeutics: principles to practice. Philadelphia: Saunders; 2009. p. 1269–94. Available at: https://www-clinicalkey-com.proxy.library.vanderbilt.edu/#!/browse/book/3-s2.0-B9781416032915X5001X.

20. Vo AA, Chaux GE, Falk JA. Transplant pharmacology. In: Lewis ML, editor. Medical management of the thoracic surgery patient. Philadelphia: Saunders; 2010.

p. 352–6. Available at: https://www-clinicalkey-com.proxy.library.vanderbilt.edu/#!/browse/book/3-s2.0-B9781416039938X00013.

21. Gotthardt DN, Bruns H, Weiss KH, et al. Current strategies for immunosuppression following liver transplantation. Langenbecks Arch Surg 2014;399(8):981–8.

22. Ruutu T, Gratwohl A, de Witte T. Prophylaxis and treatment of GVHD: EBMT–ELN working group recommendations for a standardized practice. Bone Marrow Transplant 2014;49(2):168–73.

23. Pham MX, Yee J. Cardiac transplant rejection. In: Ginsberg GH, Willard HS, editors. Genomic and personalized medicine. Tokyo: Elsevier; 2013. p. 557–71. Available at: https://www-clinicalkey-com.proxy.library.vanderbilt.edu/#!/browse/book/3-s2.0-C20091621158.

24. Molnar AO, Fergusson D, Tsampalieros AK. Generic immunosuppression in solid organ transplantation: systematic review and meta-analysis. BMJ 2015;350:h3163.

25. Klintmalm GB. Immunosuppression, generic drugs and the FDA. Am J Transplant 2011;11:1765–6.

26. Kim JM, Kwon CHD, Yun IJ, et al. A multicenter experience with generic mycophenolate mofetil conversion in stable liver transplant recipients. Ann Surg Treat Res 2014;86(4):192–8.

27. Choi SW, Reddy P. Current and emerging strategies for the prevention of graft-versus-host disease. Nat Rev Clin Oncol 2014;11:536–47.

28. Ensor CR, Trofe-Clark J, Gabardi S, et al. Generic maintenance immunosuppression in solid organ transplant recipients. Pharmacotherapy 2011;31(11):1111–29. Available at: http://onlinelibrary.wiley.com.proxy.library.vanderbilt.edu/doi/10.1592/phco.31.11.1111/abstract.

29. Penninga L, Møller CH, Gustafsson F, et al. Tacrolimus versus cyclosporine as primary immunosuppression after heart transplantation: systematic review with meta-analyses and trial sequential analyses of randomised trials. Eur J Clin Pharmacol 2010;66(12):1177–87.

30. Krau SD. Cytochrome P450 part 3: drug interactions: essential concepts and considerations. Nurs Clin North Am 2013;48(4):697–706.

31. Molina BD, Leiro MCG, Pulpón LA, et al. Incidence and risk factors for nonmelanoma skin cancer after heart transplantation. Transplant proc 2010;42(8):3001–5.

32. Feldmeyer L, Hofbauer GFL, Böni T, et al. Mammalian target of rapamycin (mTOR) inhibitors slow skin carcinogenesis, but impair wound healing. Br J Dermatol 2012;166(2):422–4.

33. Guilbeau JM. Delayed wound healing with sirolimus after liver transplant. Ann Pharmacother 2002;36(9):1391–5.

34. Kuppahally S, Al-Khaldib A, Weisshaarc D, et al. Wound healing complications with de novo sirolimus versus mycophenolate mofetil-based regimen in cardiac transplant recipients. Am J Transplant 2006;6(5p1):986–92.

35. Kaplan B, Qazi Y, Wellen JR. Strategies for management of adverse events associated with mTOR inhibitors. Transplant Rev 2014;8:126–33.

36. Soliman K, Mogadam E, Laftavi M, et al. Long-term outcomes following sirolimus conversion after renal transplantation. Immunol Invest 2014;43(8):819–28.

37. Lee RA, Gabardi S. Current trends in immunosuppressive therapies for renal transplant patients. Am J Health Syst Pharm 2012;69:1961–75.

38. Belatacept Up To Date Web site. Available at: http://www.uptodate.com.proxy.library.vanderbilt.edu/contents/belatacept-drug-information?source=search_result&search=belatacept&selectedTitle=1~16. Accessed September 13, 2015.

39. Arora S, Bhargavi T, Osadchuk L, et al. Belatacept: a new biological agent for maintenance immunosuppression in kidney transplantation. Expert Opin Biol Ther 2012;12(7):965–79.

40. Food and Drug Administration. Guidance for industry: warnings and precautions, contraindications and boxed warning sections of labeling for human prescription drug and biological products – content and format. 2011. Available at: http://www.fda.gov/downloads/Drugs/.../Guidances/ucm075096.pdf. Accessed September 12, 2015.

Vaccines and Immunization Practice

Michael D. Hogue, PharmD, FNAP[a],*, Anna E. Meador, PharmD, BCACP[a,b]

KEYWORDS

- Immunization practice • Vaccines • Vaccine-preventable diseases
- Practice guidelines

KEY POINTS

- Vaccine-preventable diseases continue to cause significant morbidity and mortality in the United States despite the availability of safe and effective vaccines.
- Adult immunization rates in the United States are well-below Healthy People 2020 targets for all vaccine-preventable diseases, and require nurses and other health care professionals to take more proactive, intentional approaches to immunizing patients.
- Immunization practice guidelines for the United States are established by the Centers for Disease Control and Prevention's Advisory Committee on Immunization Practices and published in *Morbidity and Mortality Weekly Report* at least annually, with quarterly changes occurring on action of the committee.
- Vaccines are a safe and effective intervention for protecting the public's health and should be advocated at every health care encounter.

OVERVIEW

The Institute of Medicine has conducted more than 60 studies of vaccine safety.[1] Time and again they have come to the conclusion that many public health practitioners already knew: vaccines are among of the most safe and effective public health interventions of modern times.[2] Despite decades of resoundingly positive evidence

Disclosures: Dr M.D. Hogue discloses that he is on the speaker's bureau for Pfizer, Inc and is a grant recipient from Merck. Dr A.E. Meador has no financial relationships to disclose.
Important Note: All references to vaccine schedules and vaccine information, including all information appearing in the tables, are from the 2015 Centers for Disease Control and Prevention's Advisory Committee on Immunization Practices (ACIP) current recommendations (www. cdc.gov/vaccines) unless otherwise noted. Due to the frequent changes to vaccine policy and recommendations in the United States, clinicians are strongly advised to consult the most recent vaccine schedules and ACIP recommendations before making patient care decisions.
[a] Department of Pharmacy Practice, Samford University, McWhorter School of Pharmacy, 800 Lakeshore Drive, Birmingham, AL 35229, USA; [b] Christ Health Center, 5720 1st Avenue South, Birmingham, AL 35212, USA
* Corresponding author.
E-mail address: mdhogue@samford.edu

supporting the safety of vaccines, and the documented evidence of marked decreases in the incidence and prevalence of vaccine-preventable diseases, many consumers refuse to have their children vaccinated either at all or vaccinated on time. Even more adolescent and adult patients fail to be immunized, likely due to a lack of awareness of the availability of vaccines to prevent diseases in adults, or of their relative risk of contracting the diseases the vaccines are designed to prevent.[3] Additionally, health care professionals are faced with an increasing number of vaccine products being brought to market, coupled with ever changing governmental recommendations for vaccine use. The increasing complexity in vaccine recommendation, confusion among health care professions, and a public health disconnect due to patient misperceptions has led to lower-than-desired immunization rates, particularly among adolescent and adult patients. The result: recent disease outbreaks of vaccine-preventable diseases, notably measles, which had been eliminated from United States endemic transmission for several years before its resurgence. To ensure optimal disease prevention and protection for all patients, new approaches to immunization practice are required by all members of the health care team.

IMMUNIZATION SCHEDULES

Annually (typically in February or March) the Centers for Disease Control and Prevention's (CDC's) Advisory Committee on Immunization Practices (ACIP) revises and releases new adult and childhood immunization schedules. The American Academy of Family Physicians, the American College of Physicians, The American College of Obstetricians and Gynecologists, and the American College of Nurse-Midwives have historically endorsed these schedules. The immunization schedule and a summary of changes are published in the *Annals of Internal Medicine* and are available on the CDC's Web site at www.cdc.gov/vaccines. Health care providers should become familiar with the complete recommendations. If there are any changes ACIP recommends between schedule releases, the changes are published in the *Morbidity and Mortality Weekly Report* and posted to the CDC's Web site and incorporated into the following year's schedules.[4] Updates to the adult schedule can be found at http://www.cdc.gov/vaccines/schedules/hcp/adult.html and the birth to 18 year schedule updates are available at http://www.cdc.gov/vaccines/schedules/hcp/child-adolescent.html.

When putting these schedules into practice, there are many electronic resources available to help with recommendations for providers and patients. All 50 states use a state immunization information system (IIS), frequently called registries, to track childhood vaccines. Each state designs and manages its own IIS.[5] Most IISs also can track adult immunizations. Ideally, each practice's electronic medical record will be electronically connected to the IIS to ensure seamless, streamlined data entry for each patient. Bidirectional communication allows providers to determine the current immunization status of the individual.

The CDC, via www.cdc.gov/vaccines, offers printable schedules, easy-to-read versions for parents, interactive tools for both patients and providers, as well as free laminated schedules. Because printed schedules are not updated as frequently as certain electronic resources, clinicians may decide to use digital applications (apps) for portable electronic devices to ensure the most up-to-date recommendations are being used in practice. Three reliable apps are *CDC Vaccine Schedules*, developed by the CDC; *Shots Immunizations*, developed by Society of Teachers of Family Medicine; and *ACP Immunization Advisor*, developed by the American College of Physicians. Additionally, there are many paid and free apps that are available for patients and caregivers to help remind when the series should be completed. Before recommending any app to a patient, review to ensure the information provided is accurate and complete.

VACCINE-PREVENTABLE DISEASES
Tetanus, Diphtheria, and Pertussis

Tetanus, caused by the ubiquitous anaerobic bacterium *Clostridium tetani*, is a toxin-producing pathogen that ultimately interferes with the release of neurotransmitters. This leads to a blockade of inhibitor impulses, resulting in unopposed muscle spasm and contraction. Because the disease is often associated with acute injury, the CDC has published resources for vaccination following a disaster event, as well as routine immunization following both clean minor wounds and contaminated wounds.[6,7] Diphtheria is caused by the bacterium *Corynebacterium diphtheriae*. It is most typically spread via respiratory droplets. Although diphtheria epidemics in the United States were common in the early twentieth century, endemic cases of diphtheria in the United States are largely unheard of in the postvaccine era. Due to effective vaccination strategies, there have only been 5 cases reported to the CDC in the past decade.[8,9]

Pertussis, or whooping cough, is caused by the bacterium *Bordetella pertussis*. There are at least 6 known toxins produced by the bacteria, the most serious of which can cause epiglottal swelling, paralysis of the pulmonary alveoli, and an inability to clear mucous from the lungs. These factors together lead to a characteristic whoop sound on inspiration, followed by continuous coughing that may last for several seconds or minutes. Patients can become hypoxic and, even with treatment, convalescence can take as long as 3 months. Because of waning immunity among older children, adolescents, and adults, and because these populations can be infected with either asymptomatic or mildly symptomatic disease, the United States is currently in the midst of an outbreak of pertussis that largely began in 2010. As many as 22,000 to 50,000 cases of confirmed pertussis, with dozens of deaths, mostly among infants, have been reported to the CDC each year since 2004. This number, however, is largely considered a substantial underreporting of actual disease because many adults are only mildly symptomatic or may receive treatment without laboratory confirmation of disease. Further, it seems that there may be epidemiologic changes to the bacterium itself because there have been an increasing number of cases among fully-vaccinated children and adults.[10]

The best method to prevent tetanus, diphtheria and pertussis is active immunization (**Table 1**). The ACIP recommends a 5-dose primary series with the pediatric formulation diphtheria and tetanus toxoids and acellular pertussis (DTaP) vaccine beginning at 2 months of age and continuing through 5 years of age. Multiple manufacturers provide DTaP vaccine in the commercial market. Because there are limited data on the safety, immunogenicity, and efficacy of using DTaP vaccines from different manufacturers in a mixed sequence, the ACIP generally recommends that, whenever feasible, the same brand of DTaP vaccine be used for all of the doses of the primary vaccination series.[11] However, providers who may not know or have the same brand available should administer any available DTaP vaccine to ensure a complete vaccination series. Following this primary series, it is recommended that all adolescents age 11 to 18 years receive a single booster dose of tetanus toxoid, reduced diphtheria toxoid, and acellular pertussis (Tdap) vaccine.[7]

Further, as an effort to reduce pertussis in infants, ACIP recommends using Tdap vaccine as a single dose in all pregnant women during each pregnancy ideally between the 27th and 36th weeks of gestation to maximize the maternal antibody

Table 1			
Tetanus antigen-containing vaccines			
Vaccine	ACIP Recommended Age	Dose	Schedule (if Used)
DTaP	2, 4, 6, 15–18 mo, and 4–6 y	0.5 mL	2, 4, 6, 15–18 mo, and 4–6 y
DT	Birth–19 y	0.5 mL	0, 1, 6 mo
Td	≥20 y	1.0 mL	Administered as a booster dose every 10 y after patient receives single booster of Tdap vaccine
Tdap	Ideally 11–12 y Youngest age for catch-up administration is 7 y There is no maximum age	0.5 mL	1 dose ideally 11–12 y Youngest age for catch-up administration is 7 y No maximum age All adolescents and adults should receive 1 dose of Tdap, unless there is a contraindication to receipt of a pertussis vaccine, in such case Td vaccine is recommended

Abbreviations: DT, diphtheria and tetanus toxoids; DTaP, diphtheria and tetanus toxoids and acellular pertussis; Td, tetanus and reduced diphtheria toxoids; Tdap, tetanus toxoid, reduced diphtheria toxoid, and acellular pertussis.

response and passive antibody transfer to the infant. Data modeling by the CDC indicates that Tdap vaccination during pregnancy has the potential to prevent 906 infant cases of pertussis, 462 hospitalizations, and 9 deaths.[12]

Finally, and again in response to the need to mitigate current high levels of pertussis transmission in the United States, the ACIP recommends the use of a single dose of Tdap vaccine be administered to all adults aged 19 years and older who have not previously received a dose of Tdap. Although only 1 of the 2 licensed Tdap vaccine products (Boostrix) in the United States is approved for use beyond 64 years of age, the ACIP recommends that providers not delay in immunizing patients who are unimmunized, using whichever product is available at the time the patient presents for care.[13] In addition to Tdap, there is a dual antigen vaccine, tetanus and reduced diphtheria toxoids, available for adult use. Because of waning immunity to all 3 antigens (tetanus, diphtheria, and pertussis), booster doses of tetanus antigen-containing vaccines have long been recommended for administration every 10 years. The dual antigen Td vaccine is currently recommended for use in nonpregnant adult patients who have already received 1 dose of Tdap since age 19 and who are now due for a 10 year booster dose of a tetanus-containing vaccine, or as an accelerated booster dose of tetanus-containing vaccine due to wound care guidelines in patients who have received a previous dose of Tdap vaccine.[7]

DTaP, Td, and Tdap have strong positive safety profiles. The most common adverse events are localized reactions (pain, redness at the injection site, limitation of arm movement, and arm swelling). The incidence of these reactions increases in the pediatric population with the fourth and fifth doses of the primary series, and parents should be advised that their child may experience these largely self-limiting effects. Adult patients receiving Td or Tdap vaccines may experience increased localized reactions when doses are given at intervals of less than or equal to 2 years apart. There is no significant difference in the frequency of side effects in pediatric versus adult patients, nor between DTaP (pediatric formulation) and Tdap (adolescent or adult formulation) when age-appropriate administration occurs.[7] The vaccine is contraindicated in any person who experienced a life-threatening allergic reaction after a dose of DTaP, or in a person who suffered a brain or nervous system disease within 7 days after a dose of DTaP.[7]

Measles, Mumps, and Rubella

Measles (formerly known as rubeola), mumps, and rubella (formerly known as German measles) are preventable viral illnesses. Measles and mumps viruses are both in the *Paramyxoviridae* family, whereas the rubella virus is in the *Togaviridae* family. There is no effective treatment of measles, mumps, or rubella. Medical supportive care may help relieve symptoms or prevent secondary bacterial infections. All 3 conditions are transmitted by direct contact with respiratory droplets. Measles is among the most highly contagious vaccine-preventable respiratory illnesses. The paramyxovirus can survive in room air for up to 2 hours. The incubation period is 7 to 21 days, followed by a prodome of high fever, cough, coryza (runny nose), and conjunctivitis. A few days later, Koplik spots can appear in the mouth for a brief period of time, followed by a maculopapular rash on the body. The rash can last up to 6 days. Patients are contagious for 4 days before the rash appears and for 4 days after that. This rash will affect the entire body and then slowly recede. Some complications include pneumonia, encephalitis, or death.

The measles vaccine is most effective following 2 doses.[14,15] The United States declared measles to be eliminated from endemic cases in 2000. Recent outbreaks have been due to parental refusal to vaccinate children coupled with imported measles cases entering the United States through unvaccinated individuals. As of August 21, 2015, 188 cases of measles have been reported for 2015. This is down from 2014 when 668 cases were reported.[16,17]

Mumps has an incubation period of 16 to 18 days. There is a nonspecific prodrome phase of fever, myalgia, malaise, and headache followed by parotitis (swollen salivary glands). The parotitis can be either unilateral or bilateral. Patients are contagious for about 5 days after the parotitis appears. Some patients will be completely asymptomatic or just suffer from nonspecific symptoms. The disease is fairly mild in children. Complications include meningitis, orchitis (inflamed testicles) or oophoritis (inflamed ovaries), deafness, myocarditis, and death. The vaccine is 88% effective after 2 doses. Outbreaks have occurred in the United States in recent years and are usually attributed to crowded environments where a patient has mumps.[14,18]

Rubella typically presents as a disseminated maculopapular rash of about 3 days duration. Arthralgia or arthritis are common in adult women. Complications can include encephalitis, miscarriages, stillbirth, and congenital rubella syndrome (CRS). CRS results in birth defects that range from mild to severe growth and mental retardation, as well as heart defects. Risk for CRS is highest when rubella is contracted in the first trimester of pregnancy. In 1969, when the rubella vaccine was introduced, reported cases declined 78% and CRS declined 69% in just the first 6 years. Because of effective immunization, the elimination of rubella in the United States since 2004 has been a reality. However, because of rubella's existence in other parts of the globe, the United States must maintain an active vaccination program.[14]

There are 2 vaccines approved for use in the United States that prevent measles, mumps, and rubella (MMR): trivalent (MMR-II) and a quadrivalent vaccine (ProQuad) that also protects against varicella (**Table 2**). Both are usually well tolerated with minimal adverse reactions. Common side effects include fever, transient rash or lymphadenopathy, and parotitis.[14] The Institute of Medicine has concluded that there is no causal relation between MMR vaccination and autistic spectrum disorder based on the body of evidence available.[19]

MMR vaccine is a live, attenuated, 2-dose vaccine series. If international travel is planned, children age 6 through 11 months should receive 1 dose before departure even though the vaccine is not routinely recommended in this age group due to the

Table 2 Measles, mumps, and rubella vaccines				
Vaccine	Age	Dose	Route	Schedule
MMR-II (MMR)	≥12 mo	0.5 mL	Subcutaneous	12–15 mo, 4–6 y
Proquad (MMRV)	12 mo–12 y	0.5 mL	Subcutaneous	12–15 mo, 4–6 y

potential of circulating maternal antibodies. As a result, infant travel health doses at this early age will not count toward the 2-dose series required per the ACIP recommendations. Adults born before 1957 are considered immune and do not normally require any vaccination except during outbreak situations or if the patient is a health care provider (see specific recommendations).[14] ACIP recommends that all patients born after 1957 receive 2 doses of MMR vaccine. The vaccine is contraindicated in pregnancy, immunocompromising conditions, human immunodeficiency virus (HIV) infection with CD4+ count less than 200 cells/μL, and severe allergic reaction to a vaccine component, including gelatin and neomycin. The tuberculin skin test can be administered on the same day as the MMR vaccine and, otherwise, the clinician should wait 4 weeks after the MMR vaccine to administer the test.[14,20]

ProQuad is a combination vaccine of measles, mumps, rubella and varicella (MMRV) antigen. It may be used for the primary immunization series. Contraindications are the same as MMR vaccine, with the addition of active untreated tuberculosis or febrile illness greater than 101.3°F. Because of the varicella antigen, the vaccine must be kept in the freezer. Once the vaccine has been reconstituted it may remain in the vial in a dark place in the refrigerator for up to 30 minutes before it must discarded.[21]

Haemophilus Influenza Type B

Haemophilus influenza is a bacterium, not to be confused with the viral influenza infection. The gram-negative bacterium was the leading cause of meningitis in children younger than 5 years of age as recently as the 1980s, with *H influenzae* polysaccharide serotype B (Hib) representing almost all infection.[22] A vaccine against Hib was introduced in 1990 and, since that time, incidence of Hib has decreased by 99%.[23]

There are currently 3 Food and Drug Administration (FDA)-licensed monovalent Hib-conjugate vaccines and 3 combination vaccines containing Hib-conjugate antigen available in the United States. A summary of the available vaccines is shown in **Table 3**.

Poliomyelitis

Poliomyelitis virus is perhaps among the most storied of all vaccine-preventable diseases in United States, and possibly world, history. Although many infectious diseases have caused greater numbers of infection, polio captured the world's attention because of its indiscriminant effect largely on children. Even as late as 1988, nearly 1000 children daily were infected with polio.[24] A highly transmissible disease transmitted through the fecal-oral route, children quickly develop irreversible paralysis within just a few hours following infection. With disease persisting into the late 1980s, public health officials around the globe decided to embark on an ambitious program: the attempt to eradicate polio. As of 2015, only 11 countries are not considered free of wild poliovirus (WPV) and through the first 8 months of 2015 there had been only 36 cases of WPV, all occurring in Pakistan and Afghanistan.[25]

As of 1999, only the inactivated polio vaccine (IPV), originally developed by Dr Jonas Salk in 1955, is used for active immunization in the United States. The vaccine is

Table 3
Haemophilus influenzae type B vaccines

Product	Manufacturer	Antigen Type or Composition	Primary Series Dosing Schedule
PedvaxHib	Merck & Co, Inc	PRP-OMP, monovalent	2-dose series: 2 and 4 mo Booster: 12–18 mo
ActHib	Sanofi Pasteur	PRP-T	3-dose series: 2, 4, and 6 mo Booster: 15–18 mo
Hiberix	GlaxoSmithKline	PRP-T	Approved only as a booster dose 15 mo–4 y if already had at least 1 dose of Hib vaccine
COMVAX	Merck & Co, Inc	PRP-OMP with hepatitis B antigen	3-dose series administered at 2, 4, and 12–15 mo, including those who received a birth dose of single antigen hepatitis B vaccine COMVAX should not be administered before 6 wk
Pentacel	Sanofi Pasteur	PRP-T with DTaP and polio antigens	4-dose series administered at 2, 4, 6, and 15–18 mo First dose should not be administered before 6 wk
MENHIBRIX	GlaxoSmithKline	PRP-T with *Neisseria meningitidis* serogroups C and Y antigens	4-dose series at 2, 4, 6, and 12–15 mo First dose should not be administered before 6 wk

Abbreviations: OMP, outer membrane protein; PRP, polyribosylribitol phosphate; T, tetanus toxoid conjugate.

administered via intramuscular (IM) injection to children ages 2, 4, and 6 to 18 months, and a final dose given at 4 to 5 years of age. Regardless of previous doses, the ACIP recommends 1 dose be given at age 4 years or older. An additional booster dose is recommended for international travelers of any age whose travel will take them to a country where polio has not been declared eradicated by the World Health Organization. The vaccine is very safe and effective, and no serious systemic adverse effects have ever resulted from this vaccine.[26]

Certain combination vaccines contain polio antigen. Use of combination vaccines to prevent polio is acceptable. However it is important to note that when Pentacel (DTaP-IPV/Hib) is used to provide the 4 doses of the pediatric series at 2, 4, 6, and 15 to 18 months of age, the patient will still need an additional fifth dose of IPV vaccine at 4 to 6 years of age, for a total of 5 doses of IPV-containing vaccine.[26]

Rotavirus

The CDC reports that rotavirus is the most common cause of severe gastroenteritis in infants and children. Nearly 80% of children were infected in the United States by their fifth birthday until a vaccine was introduced in 2006.[27] Two orally administered, live-attenuated rotavirus vaccines (RVs) are available on the United States market. ACIP recommends administration of either RV5 or RV1 (but not both) to all infants as a part of routine infant immunization programs. ACIP does not express a preference for a specific vaccine compared with the other; however, it is recommended that providers use the same vaccine product to complete a series. If RV5 is administered, a 3-dose series at 2, 4, and 6 months of age is recommended. If RV1 is administered, a 2-dose series at 2 and 4 months of age is recommended. Rotavirus vaccination should never be initiated in infants ages 15 weeks and 0 days or older because of insufficient safety data of the first dose in older infants. All doses must be administered no later than age 8 months and 0 days. Contraindications to the use of the vaccine include patients with a previous history of intussusception and patients with a previous history of severe allergic reaction to a previous dose.[27,28] RV1 should not be administered to patients with severe allergy to latex because there is latex in the oral applicator. RV5 does not contain latex in the dosing tube. Infants who have altered immunocompetence for any reason should only receive rotavirus vaccine after careful consultation with an immunologist or infectious disease specialist to weigh the benefits versus risks given that the vaccine is a live, attenuated vaccine and must replicate in the gastrointestinal tract to evoke an immune response. There is no precaution in preterm infants, and ACIP recommends vaccinating infants according to birth age, not gestational age.[28]

Hepatitis A Virus

Hepatitis A virus (HAV) is an RNA picornavirus that is shed in stool, making person-to-person transmission mainly through the fecal-oral route. HAV has an average incubation period of 28 days. Symptoms are similar to other hepatitis viruses and onset is abrupt and includes fever, malaise, anorexia, nausea, abdominal discomfort, dark urine, and jaundice. Patients less than 6 months of age are often asymptomatic, yet capable of spreading the virus, although most older children and adults with infections are symptomatic. Shedding is highest 2 weeks before the onset of jaundice. In children, shedding can last up to 10 weeks after onset. Infants can shed for up to 6 months. Immunoglobulin G anti-HAV appears early in the illness and remains for the patient's life and indicates lifelong immunity against the disease. The vaccine release in 1995 and the ACIP recommendation for targeted immunization in 1999 resulted in a dramatic decline in HAV rates, especially in Native American populations in which the risk was higher than other racial or ethnic groups.[29,30] After many years of targeted immunization recommendations, in 2006 ACIP recommended a 2-dose, IM hepatitis A vaccine series for all children from 1 year through 18 years of age.[29] At-risk, nonroutine, immunization of adults is recommended. Those at highest risk of HAV infection include patients with chronic liver disease, travelers to countries with high or intermediate rates of hepatitis A, and/or those who anticipate close personal contact with an international adoptee from a country with high or intermediate rates of hepatitis A during the first 60 days following arrival, and men who have sex with men (MSM).[29]

Hepatitis B virus (HBV) is a DNA virus of the *Hepadnaviridae* family and is transmitted through blood and other bodily fluids such as semen. The incubation period can range from 60 to 90 days from exposure to onset of jaundice or abnormal alanine aminotransferase (ALT) levels. However, the infection is often asymptomatic and individuals can become chronic carriers of the disease. Chronic disease patients are at an increased risk of cirrhosis and hepatocellular carcinoma, which often develop decades after initial exposure. Two vaccine products are currently available on the United States market that seem to confer lifelong immunity following a 3-dose series.[31] Hepatitis B vaccine is recommended for all children from birth through 18 years, with a birth-dose of hepatitis B vaccine before hospital discharge being the standard of care since 1990. For unvaccinated adults, the vaccine is recommended if an additional risk factor is present. These risk factors include immunocompromising conditions, HIV infection, MSM, end-stage renal disease, chronic liver disease, diabetes, and health care personnel.[32,33] Patients with diabetes benefit most from receiving the vaccine between ages 19 through 59 years of age. However, even patients who are 60 years of age or older may receive the vaccine if the patient and health care provider determine appropriate.[33]

Hepatitis B vaccine is recombinant hepatitis B surface antigen (HBsAG) and marketed as Recombivax HB or Engerix-B, both administered IM. For adolescents ages 11 through 15 years there are 2 options for Recombivax-HB: 0.5 mL given at the regular series or 1.0 mL given at 0 and 4 to 6 months. Engerix-B can only be given in a 3-dose series at 0, 1, and 6 months and is not approved for 2-dose adolescent schedule. Combination vaccines that contain hepatitis B antigen may be preferred (not including the birth dose) when other vaccine antigens are also indicated (eg, in pediatric patients). Consult the current ACIP General Practice Recommendations for more information about use of combination vaccines[34] (**Table 4**).

Varicella (Chickenpox) and Herpes Zoster (Shingles)

Varicella zoster virus is an aerosolized virus transmitted primarily through respiratory droplets to susceptible individuals, although direct contact with vesicular fluid of patients with active (acute) lesions of either varicella (chickenpox) or zoster (shingles) is also a known method of transmission. Following exposure to the virus, infected individuals are contagious within 1 to 2 days before the onset of the classic chickenpox rash, which is typically 14 to 16 days following exposure. Most patients are contagious until all lesions have crusted, or about 1 week after the onset of rash.[35] On resolution of chickenpox infection, the virus remains dormant in the sensory-nerve ganglia of the dorsal spine, remaining largely in check by a functional, normal immune system for the remainder of life. However, as persons age, experience extreme stress of any cause, or develop an altered immunocompetence (either acutely or chronically), the development of a painful, zoster rash along 1 or more dermatomes may occur. Known as shingles, zoster can be a serious and debilitating illness. A full range of neurologic issues are possible; however, the most common and debilitating consequence is a chronic pain syndrome known as postherpetic neuralgia (PHN). Hallmarked by pain that lasts for weeks, months, or years following the resolution of zoster rash, the PHN can disrupt sleep, mood, work, and activities of daily living.[36]

Prevention of primary varicella infection has been possible because a vaccine was licensed and recommended for routine use in 1995. Varicella vaccine (Varivax) must be frozen and protected from light. It must be reconstituted using a manufacturer-supplied diluent not more than 30 minutes before being administered. The vaccine is administered in a 2-dose series to all children 15 to 18 months and 4 to 5 years of age. Quadrivalent MMRV vaccine may be used instead of single antigen vaccine for either or both doses. The vaccine is contraindicated in patients with immunocompromising conditions, iatrogenic immunosuppression, during pregnancy, and in those who have a history of anaphylactic reactions to gelatin, neomycin, or any other vaccine component.[35]

Table 4 Hepatitis A and Hepatitis B			
Vaccine	**Age**	**Dose**	**Schedule**
Vaqta or Havrix (hepatitis A)	12 mo–18 y	0.5 mL	Vaqta: 0, 6–18 mo
	≥19	1.0 mL	Havrix: 0, 6–12 mo
Recombivax HB or Engerix-B (hepatitis B)	Birth–19 y	0.5 mL	Recombivax HB: 0, 1, 6 mo
	≥20 y	1.0 mL	Engerix-B: 0, 1, 6 mo
Recombivax HB (hepatitis B dialysis)	≥20 y	1.0 mL	0, 1, 6 mo
Engerix-B (hepatitis B) for dialysis patients	≥20 y	1.0 mL	2 doses given at 0, 1, 2, and 6-mo
Twinrix (hepatitis A and B)	≥18 y	1.0 mL	0, 1, 6 mo or 0, 7, 21–30 d Booster: 1 y

Varicella zoster vaccine (Zostavax) is FDA-approved for use in adult patients 50 years of age and older to prevent shingles, although ACIP recommends the use of the vaccine in patients aged 60 years and older. The zoster vaccine, which is markedly different in antigen content from the pediatric varicella vaccine and should never be given to pediatric patients, requires the same storage and handling, precautions, and contraindications for use as the varicella vaccine.[37] It is currently recommended as a single dose for all adult patients older than age 60 years, with no booster dose currently recommended. Because the vaccine is a live, attenuated vaccine, the CDC, FDA, and manufacturer all strongly advise that the vaccine should not be transported between providers and should be administered by the clinician who stores the vaccine.[36]

Pneumococcal Vaccines

Streptococcus pneumoniae (pneumococcus) is among the most prevalent vaccine-preventable infections among adults in the United States The CDC estimates that pneumococcus is responsible for 4 million illness episodes, 445,000 hospitalizations, and 22,000 deaths annually.[38] Despite availability of vaccine in the United States to prevent pneumococcus since the 1970s, immunization rates among high-risk adults, including those with age-based risk, remain low.[38]

In 2015, the ACIP recommended a revised strategy for immunization of adult patients older than 65 years of age against pneumococcal disease.[39] A summary of the recommendations for the 2 pneumococcal vaccines currently available is given in **Table 5**.

Human Papillomavirus

Human papillomavirus (HPV), the most common sexually transmitted infection, is a DNA papillomavirus that resides in the epithelium. Patients should ideally be immunized before any sexual activity. Although many patients are asymptomatic, HPV is the primary cause of both genital warts and cervical cancers depending on the infecting serotype.[42] In addition to cervical cancers, vulvar, vaginal, penile, anal, and oropharyngeal cancers are also caused by HPV. The high-risk serotypes 16 and 18 cause about 64% of these cancers and serotypes 31, 33, 45, 52, and 58 cause about 10% of these cancers. About 75% of noncancerous high-grade cervical lesions are also caused by these serotypes.[43] Serotypes 6 and 11 and are responsible for more than 90% of genital warts. HPV vaccines are recommended for all female patients ages 9 to 26 years and all male patients ages 9 through 21 years. Immunocompromised men and MSM older than age 21 are recommended to receive either the quadrivalent or 9-serotype vaccine through age 26. The bivalent vaccine is not approved for male patients of any age.[42,43]

Human Papillomavirus Vaccines			
Vaccine	ACIP Age Recommendations	Approved Ages	HPV Types Included
Cervarix (HPV2)	Female patients: 9–26 y	Female patients: 9–25 y	16, 18
Gardasil (HPV4)	Female patients: 9–26 y	Female and male patients: 9–26 y	6, 11, 16, 18
Gardasil 9 (HPV9)	Male patients: 9–21 y	Female patients: 9–26 y Male patients: 9–15 y	6, 11, 16, 18, 31, 33, 45, 52, 58

Meningococcal

Meningococcal disease is a bacterial infection caused by *Neisseria meningitidis*. It is spread through contact with respiratory droplets and can present as meningitis,

Table 5
Pneumococcal vaccines and recommendations

Vaccine	Dose, Route	ACIP Recommendation	Special Considerations
Pneumococcal polysaccharide vaccine, 23 valent, PPSV-23 (Pneumovax-23)	0.5 mL, IM or subcutaneous	• 1 dose for all persons ≥65 y at least 1 y after PCV-13 • 2 doses, separated by 5 y, in high-risk individuals 6–64 y and following 1 dose of PCV-13 • 1 dose in patients 19–64 y with certain chronic medical conditions	• ACIP recommends a 1-y interval between PPSV-23 and PCV-13 in patients >65 y • PPSV-23 can follow PCV-13 at an 8-wk minimum interval in patients who are immunocompromised
Pneumococcal conjugate vaccine, 13 valent, PCV-13 (Prevnar-13)	0.5 mL, IM	• 4-dose pediatric series at 2, 4, 6, and 12–15 mo • 1 dose in patients ≥65 y • 1 dose in patients 19–64 with immuno-compromising conditions	Regardless of age of administration, in patients who have already received PPSV-23, PCV-13 should be administered 1 y later

For a complete listing of conditions the ACIP considers immunocompromising and high risk for pneumococcal disease, and for the list of chronic medical conditions indicating the need for pneumococcal vaccination, see Refs.[40,41] In addition, ACIP recommends specific timing and spacing of vaccine doses in patients 65 years and older depending on previous vaccination history. Consult Ref.[39] for more information.

bacteremia, or bacteremic pneumonia. Meningitis is the most common presentation; its symptoms include headache, fever, stiff neck, nausea, vomiting, photophobia, and/or altered mental status. Adolescents and young adults are typically the population with the highest percentage of asymptomatic carriers. The 6 major serogroups of meningococcal virus are A, B, C, W-135, X, and Y. Serogroups B, C, and Y cause most meningococcal disease in the United States. However, in persons ages 11 and older, the most prevalent serogroups are C, Y, and W and they account for 73% of cases.[44] Internationally, serogroup A is the most prevalent; however, serogroups C, X, and W also occur and may be common in some countries.[45] ACIP recommendations for meningococcal vaccines are somewhat complex with the addition of serogroup B vaccine in 2014. These recommendations are based on the serogroup coverage provided.

Vaccine	Serogroups	FDA-Approved Ages	Dose	Route	Schedule
Menomune (MPSV4)	A, C, W, and Y	≥2 y	0.5 mL	Subcutaneous	1 dose, booster at 5 y
Menactra (MenACWY-D)	A, C, W, and Y	9 mo–55 y	0.5 mL	IM	Single dose except in highest risk patients
Menveo (MenACWY-CRM)	A, C, W, and Y	2 mo–55 y	0.5 mL	IM	Single dose except in highest risk patients
MenHibrix (HiB-MenCY)	C and Y	6 wk–18 mo	0.5 mL	IM	2, 4, 6, 12–15 mo
Trumenba (MenB-FHbp)	B	10–25 y	0.5 mL	IM	0, 2, 6 mo
Bexsero (MenB-4C)	B	10–25 y	0.5 mL	IM	0 and 1–6 mo

There are 6 meningococcal vaccine products on the market today. They can be divided into 3 categories based on serogroup coverage. The first category is quadrivalent vaccines covering serogroups A, C, W-135, and Y (MPSV4 and MenACWY). The second category contains only 1 bivalent vaccine that covers serogroups C and Y (MenCY). The final category for vaccines contains only serogroup B coverage (MenB).[44]

Vaccination against serotypes A, C, W, and Y are recommended for all children aged 11 through 18 years and children ages 2 months through 10 years who are at increased risk for meningococcal disease.[44]

Those at highest risk of meningococcal disease include patients who are asplenic, have persistent complement component deficiency, and those who travel to an endemic region. Microbiologists who may work with the bacteria in a laboratory setting, first-year college students living in residence halls, and military recruits who have had not had a dose on or after their 16th birthday should be immunized with the quadrivalent vaccine.[44] The MenB vaccines are recommended for patients ages 10 and up with persistent complement component deficiencies, anatomic or functional asplenia, microbiologists, and persons at increased risk during serogroup B outbreak. MenB vaccine is currently not recommended for routine use among college students or military recruits.[46]

Influenza

Influenza virus is a respiratory illness seen most commonly in the United States from late fall to early spring. There are 2 types of influenza that cause human disease: influenza A and B. Influenza A is then subcategorized based on 2 surface antigens, hemagglutinin (HA) and neuraminidase (NA). Influenza A is known to undergo antigenic drift, frequently leading to seasonal epidemics and the need for different vaccines each year. Trivalent formulations of influenza inactivated vaccine (IIV)-3 contain 2 influenza A strains (H1N1 and H3N2) and 1 influenza B strain. The quadrivalent, IIV4, contains the same as IIV3 with an extra influenza B strain.[47] Each year the types of influenza strains included in influenza vaccines are predicted using models from the flu season in China to predict what will be seen in the United States. With this in mind, the efficacy of the flu vaccine changes each year. Despite the change, ACIP recommends that all patient ages 6 months or older receive an influenza vaccine each flu season. Most patients will require only 1 dose of influenza vaccine each influenza season. The patients who require 2 doses are those ages 6 months to 8 years who have not previously received 2 doses since July 1, 2015. The 2 doses do not need to be in the same year. The second dose is to be administered at least 4 weeks after the first dose.[47]

There are 2 types of influenza vaccine: live, attenuated influenza vaccine (LAIV) and IIV. The IIV is then divided into 4 formulations: IIV3, IIV4, cell culture-based trivalent (ccIIV3), and recombinant trivalent (RIV3). The LAIV is currently only available in the quadrivalent formulation (LAIV4).[47] See **Table 6** for all formulations, doses, and age indications. All formulations except intranasal vaccine recommend that the vials be shaken before administration. Most formulations should be administered IM in the deltoid or anterolateral area of the thigh depending on the age of the patient; however, there is a product designed for intradermal administration, a product for intranasal administration, and a product approved for administration using a needle-free jet injector.[47] Clinicians should familiarize themselves with the individual products available within his or her practice before administering the vaccine. All influenza vaccines carry a contraindication for severe allergic reaction to any component of the vaccine, including eggs. One product, Flublok, is free of egg protein.[48] **Table 6** lists the FDA-approved influenza vaccines in 2015.

Table 6
Influenza vaccines, United States 2015

Trade Name	Type	FDA Age Indications	Dose
Fluarix Quadrivalent	IIV4	≥3 y	0.5 mL
FluLaval Quadrivalent	IIV4	≥3 y	0.5 mL
Flu Zone Quadrivalent	IIV4	6–35 mo	0.25 mL
		≥36 mo	0.5 mL
		≥6 mo	0.25–0.5 mL
Fluzone Quadrivalent Intradermal	IIV4	18–64 y	0.1 mL
FluMist Quadrivalent Intranasal	LAIV4	2–49 y	0.2 mL
Alfuria	IIV3	≥9 y	0.5 mL
Fluvirin	IIV3	≥4 y	0.5 mL
Fluzone	IIV3	≥6 mo	0.25–0.5 mL
Flucelvax	ccIIV3	≥18 y	0.5 mL
Fluzone High-Dose	IIV3	≥65 y	0.5 mL
FluBlok	RIV3	≥18 y	0.5 mL

SUMMARY

Vaccine recommendations for the United States are comprehensive and cover the life span from birth through end of life. Immunizations should be a routine component of every medical care encounter, regardless of setting. ACIP recommendations for vaccination change frequently and new vaccine products come to market nearly every year. As a result, staying current on the latest recommendations for vaccines and their use in patients can be a daunting challenge for clinicians. Although this article is comprehensive in its overview of available vaccine products, there are many patient-specific considerations which must be taken into account that are beyond the scope of this article. It is imperative that the clinician receive in-depth and proper training such as is available through the CDC and the National Foundation for Infectious Diseases (www.nfid.org) in the use of vaccines in clinical practice to ensure optimal patient outcomes and eliminate missed opportunities for disease prevention.

REFERENCES

1. Healthy people 2020 Web site. Available at: www.healthypeople.gov/2020/topics-objectives/topic/immunization-and-infectious-diseases. Accessed August 30, 2015.
2. Committee on the Assessment of Studies of Health Outcomes Related to the Recommended Childhood Immunization Schedule. The childhood immunization schedule and safety: stakeholder concerns, scientific evidence, and future studies. Washington, DC: Institute of Medicine of the National Academies. National Academies Press; 2013.
3. Luthy KE, Thompson KE, Beckstrand RL, et al. Perception of safety, importance and effectiveness of vaccinations among urban school employees in Utah. J Am Assoc Nurse Pract 2015;27(6):313–20.
4. Immunization schedules Web page. Centers for Disease Control and Prevention Web site. Available at: http://www.cdc.gov/vaccines/schedules/index.html. Accessed August 30, 2015.
5. Immunization information systems state/territory/city registry staff contacts Web page. Centers for Disease Control and Prevention Web site. Available

at: http://www.cdc.gov/vaccines/programs/iis/contacts-registry-staff.html. Accessed August 30, 2015.

6. Centers for Disease Control and Prevention. Recommendations for postexposure interventions to prevent infection with hepatitis B virus, hepatitis C virus, or human immunodeficiency virus, and tetanus in persons wounded during bombings and other mass-casualty events—United States, 2008. MMWR Recomm Rep 2008; 57(RR06):1–19.

7. Centers for Disease Control and Prevention. Updated recommendations for use of tetanus toxoid, reduced diphtheria toxoid and acellular pertussis (Tdap) vaccine from the Advisory Committee on Immunization Practices, 2010. MMWR Morb Mortal Wkly Rep 2011;60(01):13–5.

8. Centers for Disease Control and Prevention. Summary of notifiable diseases—United States, 2012. MMWR Morb Mortal Wkly Rep 2014;61(53):1–121.

9. Diphtheria Web page for clinicians. Centers for Disease Control and Prevention. Available at: http://www.cdc.gov/diphtheria/clinicians.html. Accessed August 5, 2015.

10. Pertussis/whooping cough 2014 case definition. National Notifiable Diseases Surveillance System (NNDSS) Web page. Centers for Disease Control and Prevention. Available at: http://wwwn.cdc.gov/nndss/script/casedef.aspx?CondYrID=950&DatePub=1/1/2014. Accessed August 5, 2015.

11. Advisory Committee on Immunization Practices. Use of diphtheria toxoid-tetanus toxoid-acellular pertussis vaccine as a five-dose series: supplemental recommendations of the Advisory Committee on Immunization Practices. MMWR Recomm Rep 2000;49(RR13):1–8.

12. Centers for Disease Control and Prevention. Updated recommendations for the use of tetanus toxoid, reduced diphtheria toxoid, and acellular pertussis vaccine (Tdap) in pregnant women—Advisory Committee on Immunization Practices (ACIP), 2012. MMWR Morb Mortal Wkly Rep 2013;62(07):131–5.

13. Centers for Disease Control and Prevention. Updated recommendations for use of tetanus toxoid, reduced diphtheria toxoid, and acellular pertussis (Tdap) vaccine in adults aged 65 years and older–Advisory Committee on Immunization Practices (ACIP), 2012. MMWR Morb Mortal Wkly Rep 2012;61(25):468–70.

14. Centers for Disease Control and Prevention. Prevention of measles, rubella, congenital rubella syndrome, and mumps, 2013: summary recommendations of the Advisory Committee on Immunization Practices (ACIP). MMWR Recomm Rep 2013;62(4):1–34.

15. Measles (rubeola): for healthcare professionals. Centers for Disease Control and Prevention Web site. 2015. Available at: http://www.cdc.gov/measles/hcp/index.html. Accessed August 27, 2015.

16. Measles (rubeola): measles cases and outbreaks. Centers for Disease Control and Prevention Web site. Available at: http://www.cdc.gov/measles/cases-outbreaks.html. Accessed August 27, 2015.

17. Clemmons NS, Gastanaduy PA, Fiebelkorn AP, et al. Measles—United States, January 4–April 2, 2105. MMWR Morb Mortal Wkly Rep 2015;64(14):373–6.

18. Mumps cases and outbreaks Web page. Centers for Disease Control and Prevention Web site. Available at: http://www.cdc.gov/mumps/outbreaks.html. Accessed August 30, 2015.

19. Immunization Safety Review Committee. Immunization safety review: vaccines and autism. Washington, DC: Institute of Medicine; 2004. Available at: http://www.nap.edu/catalog/10997.html. Accessed August 30, 2015.

20. MMR-II [package insert]. Whitehouse Station, NJ: Merck & Co, Inc; 2014.

21. Proquad [package insert]. Whitehouse Station, NJ: Merck & Co, Inc; 2014.
22. Advisory Committee on Immunization Practices. Prevention and control of *Haemophilus influenzae* type b disease: Recommendations of the Advisory Committee on Immunization Practices. Centers for Disease Control and Prevention. MMWR Recomm Rep 2014;63(RR01):1–14.
23. *Haemophilus influenzae* disease (including Hib) Web page. Centers for Disease Control and Prevention Web site. Available at: http://www.cdc.gov/hi-disease/clinicians.html. Accessed August 18, 2015.
24. Brooks T. The end of polio? Behind the scenes of the campaign to vaccinate every child on the planet. Washington, DC: American Public Health Association; 2007.
25. Polio global eradication initiative Web page. World Health Organization Web site. Available at: http://www.polioeradication.org/Dataandmonitoring/Poliothisweek.aspx. Accessed August 20, 2015.
26. Advisory Committee on Immunization Practices, Centers for Disease Control and Prevention. Updated recommendations of the Advisory Committee on Immunization Practices regarding routine poliovirus vaccination. MMWR Morb Mortal Wkly Rep 2009;58(30):829–30.
27. Cortese MM, Parashar UD, Centers for Disease Control and Prevention (CDC). Prevention of rotavirus gastroenteritis among infants and children: recommendations of the Advisory Committee on Immunization Practices (ACIP). MMWR Recomm Rep 2009;58(RR02):1–25.
28. Centers for Disease Control and Prevention. Addition of history of intussusception as a contraindication for rotavirus vaccination. MMWR Morb Mortal Wkly Rep 2011;60(41):1427.
29. Centers for Disease Control and Prevention. Prevention of hepatitis A through active or passive immunization: recommendations of the Advisory Committee on Immunization Practices (ACIP). MMWR Recomm Rep 2006;55(RR–7):1–23.
30. Centers for Disease Control and Prevention. Updated recommendations from the Advisory Committee on Immunization Practices (ACIP) for use of hepatitis A vaccine in close contacts of newly arriving international adoptees. MMWR Morb Mortal Wkly Rep 2009;58(36):1006–7.
31. Centers for Disease Control and Prevention. A comprehensive immunization strategy to eliminate transmission of hepatitis B virus infection in the United States: recommendations of the Advisory Committee on Immunization Practices (ACIP); Part 1: Immunization of infants, children, and adolescents. MMWR Recomm Rep 2005;54(RR–16):1–30.
32. Centers for Disease Control and Prevention. A comprehensive immunization strategy to eliminate transmission of hepatitis B virus infection in the United States: recommendations of the Advisory Committee on Immunization Practices (ACIP); Part II: Immunization of adults. MMWR Recomm Rep 2006;55(RR–16):1–29.
33. Ahmed F, Ternte JL, Campos-Outcalt D, et al. Use of Hepatitis B vaccination for adults with diabetes mellitus: recommendations of the Advisory Committee on Immunization Practices (ACIP). MMWR Morb Mortal Wkly Rep 2011;60(50):1709–11.
34. Centers for Disease Control and Prevention. General recommendations on immunization: recommendations of the Advisory Committee on Immunization Practices (ACIP). MMWR Recomm Rep 2011;60(RR02):1–60.
35. Advisory Committee on Immunization Practices. Prevention of varicella: recommendations of ACIP. MMWR Recomm Rep 2007;56(RR–04):1–40.

36. Advisory Committee on Immunization Practices. Prevention of herpes zoster: recommendations of the ACIP. MMWR Recomm Rep 2008;57(05):1–30.
37. Zostavax [Package Insert]. Whitehouse Station, NJ: Merck & Co, Inc; 2006.
38. Cos CM. Link-Gelles R. Chapter 11: pneumococcal. In: Manual for the surveillance of vaccine-preventable diseases. Atlanta (GA): Centers for Disease Control and Prevention. Available at: http://www.cdc.gov/vaccines/pubs/surv-manual/chpt11-pneumo.html. Accessed August 30, 2015.
39. Centers for Disease Control and Prevention. Use of 13-valent pneumococcal conjugate vaccine and 23-valent pneumococcal polysaccharide vaccine among adults aged ≥65 years: recommendations of the Advisory Committee on Immunization Practices (ACIP). MMWR Morb Mortal Wkly Rep 2014;63(37):822–5.
40. Centers for Disease Control and Prevention. Use of 13-valent pneumococcal conjugate vaccine and 23-valent pneumococcal polysaccharide vaccine among children aged 6–18 years with immunocompromising conditions: recommendations of the Advisory Committee on Immunization Practices (ACIP). MMWR Morb Mortal Wkly Rep 2013;62(25):521–4.
41. Centers for Disease Control and Prevention. Use of 13-valent pneumococcal conjugate vaccine and 23-valent pneumococcal polysaccharide vaccine for adults with immunocompromising conditions: recommendations of the Advisory Committee on Immunization Practices (ACIP). MMWR Morb Mortal Wkly Rep 2012;61(40):816–9.
42. Markowitz LE, Dunne EF, Saraiya M, et al. Human papillomavirus vaccination: recommendations of the Advisory Committee on Immunization Practices (ACIP). MMWR Recomm Rep 2014;63(5):1–29.
43. Petrosky E, Bocchini JA, Hariri S, et al. Use of 9-valent human papillomavirus (HPV) vaccine: updated HPV vaccination recommendations of the Advisory Committee on Immunization Practices. MMWR Morb Mortal Wkly Rep 2015;64(11):300–4.
44. Centers for Disease Control and Prevention. Prevention and control of meningococcal disease: recommendations of the Advisory Committee on Immunization Practices (ACIP). MMWR Recomm Rep 2013;62(2):1–28.
45. MacNeil JR, Meyer SA. Meningococcal disease. In: Brunette GW, editor. CDC health information for international travel, 2016. New York: Oxford University Press; 2015. p. 263–8.
46. Folaranmi T, Rubin L, Martin SW, et al. Use of serogroups B meningococcal vaccines in persons aged ≥10 years at increased risk for serogroups B meningococcal disease: recommendations of Advisory Committee on Immunization Practices, 2015. MMWR Morb Mortal Wkly Rep 2015;64(22):608–12.
47. Grohskopf LA, Sokolow LZ, Olsen SJ, et al. Prevention and control of influenza with vaccines: recommendations of the Advisory Committee on Immunization Practices, United States, 2015-16 influenza season. MMWR Morb Mortal Wkly Rep 2015;64(30):818–25.
48. Flublok [package insert]. Meriden, CT: Protein Sciences Corporation; 2015.

Index

Note: Page numbers of article titles are in **boldface** type.

Nurs Clin N Am 51 (2016) 137–149
http://dx.doi.org/10.1016/S0029-6465(16)00017-7
0029-6465/16/$ – see front matter © 2016 Elsevier Inc. All rights reserved.

nursing.theclinics.com

Moving?

Make sure your subscription moves with you!

To notify us of your new address, find your **Clinics Account Number** (located on your mailing label above your name), and contact customer service at:

Email: journalscustomerservice-usa@elsevier.com

800-654-2452 (subscribers in the U.S. & Canada)
314-447-8871 (subscribers outside of the U.S. & Canada)

Fax number: 314-447-8029

Elsevier Health Sciences Division
Subscription Customer Service
3251 Riverport Lane
Maryland Heights, MO 63043

ELSEVIER

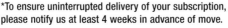